Supervising and Assessing Student Nurses and Midwives in Clinical Practice

A PRACTICAL GUIDE

Supervising and Assessing Student Nurses and Midwives in Clinical Practice

A PRACTICAL GUIDE

Jacqueline Leigh
Professor of Nurse Education Practice,
University of Salford

and

Debbie Roberts
Professor and Head of Health and Social Care Cluster,
University of Chester, Shrewsbury

ISBN 9781908625878

First published in 2021 by Lantern Publishing Ltd

Lantern Publishing Ltd, The Old Hayloft, Vantage Business Park, Bloxham Rd, Banbury OX16 9UX, UK

www.lanternpublishing.com

British Library Cataloguing in Publication Data

A catalogue record for this book is available from the British Library

The authors and publisher have made every attempt to ensure the content of this book is up to date and accurate. However, healthcare knowledge and information is changing all the time so the reader is advised to double-check any information in this text on drug usage, treatment procedures, the use of equipment, etc. to confirm that it complies with the latest safety recommendations, standards of practice and legislation, as well as local Trust policies and procedures. Students are advised to check with their tutor and/or practice supervisor before carrying out any of the procedures in this textbook.

Typeset by Medlar Publishing Solutions Pvt Ltd, India

Cover design by AM Graphic Design

Printed in the UK

Last digit is the print number: 10 9 8 7 6 5 4 3 2

CONTENTS

ABOUT THE AUTHORS

Kisma Anderson is a practice education facilitator/locality coach. Kisma is passionate about working with people to recognise and develop their skills, setting and achieving goals and recognising their strengths for career development and/or personal development. Kisma is a level 5 coach and mentor with a wealth of experience supporting staff and learners from a wide range of healthcare, social care and education environments to enable them to realise their potential and develop and/or plan and implement changes to address issues that are important to them. Kisma takes a very structured, practical approach and believes good communication and organisation enable her to offer the best support for the people with whom she works.

Joanna Barlow is a clinical specialist radiographer based at the Clatterbridge Cancer Centre, Wirral, UK. Joanna qualified as a diagnostic radiographer in 2005 with the University of Wales, Bangor, and undertook formal postgraduate education in nuclear medicine and hybrid imaging in 2009 through Salford University. In 2018, she took up a university lectureship at the School of Health Sciences, Bangor University, where she joined the lecturing and clinical tutor team to support students on the highest-ranking diagnostic radiography degree programme in the UK, and where she gained her postgraduate certificate in higher education. Joanna is a highly experienced radiographer having gained a wealth of experience working across the UK and across a broad spectrum of medical imaging modalities. Joanna has a strong background within all general X-ray areas and has specialist training and expertise in areas such as trauma, forensic radiography, theatre radiography, CT scanning, interventional and cardiac imaging as well as nuclear imaging including PETCT. In addition to her clinical and teaching expertise, Joanna is also an experienced researcher engaged with primary clinical research and clinical trials.

Dr Elaine Beaumont is a psychotherapist who specialises in cognitive behavioural therapy (CBT), compassion focused therapy (CFT) and eye movement desensitisation and reprocessing (EMDR). Elaine works with a range of organisations and charities primarily working with people who have experienced either primary or secondary trauma. Elaine is also a part-time lecturer at the University of Salford. Her academic interests focus on therapeutic interventions for trauma, compassion in healthcare and the importance of practitioner self-care. Elaine is passionate about helping people in the healthcare professions (emergency service personnel, midwives, nurses and therapists) cultivate compassion for their own suffering. Elaine's work with midwives suggests that bearing witness to the suffering of others can take its toll. Self-critical judgement, low levels of self-compassion, symptoms of stress, compassion fatigue, trauma and burnout can all have a negative impact on individuals who bear witness to trauma. Elaine's research explores the impact compassionate mind training (CMT) has on people working in the helping professions and on people who have experienced trauma. Elaine provides workshops regarding mental health, compassion and wellbeing for the NHS and a variety of organisations, and her research has been presented worldwide. Elaine co-authored *The Compassionate Mind Workbook: A step-by-step guide to developing your compassionate self* in 2017, *The Kindness Workbook: Creative and compassionate ways to boost your wellbeing* in 2020, and *The Compassionate Mind* app.

Dr Leigh Campbell qualified as a physiotherapist 20 years ago and has since worked within a range of settings and service user groups within neurological physiotherapy to develop into advanced practitioner roles in both Salford and North Wales. Leigh completed various clinical MSc modules at the University of Nottingham before completing a professional doctorate exploring the experiences of physiotherapy for people with multiple sclerosis last year at the University of Wales. She currently works as an assistant professor and lecturer in neurological physiotherapy at the University of Nottingham. Multidisciplinary and integrated team working have always been pivotal to her practice, learning and teaching, and she holds the view that this optimises best practice being delivered both to individuals and within wider healthcare. Leigh feels lucky to have worked with many people who have been willing to share their knowledge and experience and strives to continually learn from this and always do the same for others.

Hannah Dixon is a registered nurse qualifying with a first class BN (Hons) in Adult Nursing from the University of Chester. While at university Hannah undertook the role of peer mentor and peer trainer, also having involvement in the co-design and implementation of the new induction programme for nursing students. Hannah was an active member of the Student Empowerment Group and alongside this Hannah has also presented her work as an undergraduate at both national and international conferences. Since qualifying Hannah has worked in the clinical speciality of digestive diseases as a surgical nurse and in 2020 was part of the COVID palliative support team at Warrington and Halton teaching hospitals.

Leah Greene (MRes, BSc (Hons), PGCert HEPR, FHEA) is a senior lecturer in simulation-based education, Department of Nursing and Department of Health Professions, Manchester Metropolitan University, Manchester, England. She has a vast amount of experience of providing accessible, supportive simulation experiences to enhance skills and develop confident, competent healthcare personnel. She is particularly interested in using technology, simulation and mixed realities to enhance teaching and learning. She works closely with service users and carers to integrate their experiences of healthcare into realistic simulation scenarios. Leah is the Programme Lead for the Level 7 Simulation and Technology Enhanced Learning (STEL) in Healthcare PGCert programme. She has experience of project management and simulation strategy development. She was co-project lead and principal investigator for the previous Simulated Patient Train-The-Trainer (3TSP) and Train-The-Simulated Patient (2TSP) projects, funded by NHS Health Education England (HEE). Leah now runs the Simulated Patient Project for the North West Simulation Education Network (NWSEN) on behalf of HEE, training simulated patient trainers (SPTs) to deploy and integrate the Simulated Patient Common Framework and Checklist into their own organisations, enabling them to train their own cohorts of SPTs. She is currently co-investigator for the M-Care project, also funded by HEE, which is investigating the use of simulation and mixed realities to inspire young people to consider health and social care careers in the future.

Professor Caroline J. Hollins Martin (PhD, MPhil, BSc, RM, RGN, MBPsS, senior fellow HEA) has had a long career working in the area of women's health, with a specific focus upon psychological issues surrounding pregnancy and childbirth. Caroline's background has encompassed a career in women's reproductive health that spans 35 years. The first 11 years of her career were spent working as a full-time clinical midwife in Ayrshire Central Hospital (Irvine), which is now known as the Ayrshire Maternity Unit (Kilmarnock), and is based in the west of Scotland (UK). The other 24 years of Caroline's working life have been spent teaching and researching women's reproductive health within universities. To date, she has worked for the University of the West of Scotland (UWS), University of York, University of Manchester, Glasgow Caledonian University, University of Salford and Edinburgh Napier University (5 years). Caroline is a Nursing and Midwifery Council (NMC) registered midwife and lecturer/ practice educator, and also a graduate and postgraduate in psychology and Member of the British Psychological Society (MBPsS). Caroline's research interests lie in social psychology that relates to women's reproductive health, with earlier work relating to hierarchies within organisations and their effects upon decision-making and providing choice and control to childbearing women. More recently focus has shifted to developing useful tools for maternal health practitioners to use in clinical practice, such as the Birth Satisfaction Scale-Revised (BSS-R), which has been validated to assess mothers' perceptions of their birth experience. Other research interests lie in perinatal bereavement, compassionate mindfulness therapy (CMT) and PTSD.

Professor Jacqueline Leigh is a Professor of Nurse Education Practice at the University of Salford and is a registered nurse. Her contributions to learning and teaching positively influence the University of Salford activities and have had national and international reach. An advocate for interprofessional, evidence-based education, teaching and learning, Jacqueline has significant experience in developing and evaluating innovative curricula that meet workforce needs in health and social care. She leads the Educational Research and Scholarship Cluster at the University of Salford and works across the North West of England creating opportunities for the development of the healthcare workforce around interprofessional supervision and assessment in clinical practice. Jacqueline's expertise in nurse education practice is recognised at the highest level, receiving multiple learning and teaching awards including UK/International Advance HE Principal Fellow, National Teaching Fellow, Collaborative Award for Teaching Excellence, and multiple University of Salford Vice Chancellor Distinguished Teaching Awards. As an experienced NHS Leadership Academy Healthcare Leadership 360 Feedback Facilitator, Jacqueline coaches and mentors senior healthcare leaders as part of the North West Leadership Academy mentoring scheme. She is on the editorial board of the *British Journal of Nursing* and deputy chair of Healthwatch Salford.

Anne Medcalf (RN, PGCE and practice educator/lecturer, BSc Nursing Practice, MSc Professional Practice Development) qualified as a registered adult nurse in 1998 and her clinical background is in theatre and critical care nursing. Moving into education as a clinical facilitator for nursing students and then her current multiprofessional role as a practice education facilitator at the Northern Care Alliance (NCA), Anne is passionate about learning in practice, and quality clinical placements being available for all healthcare students. Anne is the synergy lead for three of the care organisations in the National Care Agency working to set up the placement model and implement a coaching approach in practice areas. Training all members of staff on 11 varied ward areas to use a different approach to supporting and assessing students in practice by developing the use of coaching conversations has had a positive impact on both student learning and recruitment of newly qualified nurses.

Peggy Murphy is a senior lecturer in adult nursing at the University of Chester. She has nursing experience in acute medicine and also cardiothoracic intensive care and has worked as a registered nurse in both the UK and Australia. She became a nurse lecturer in 2003 and developed an interest in working with students as partners to enhance inclusive practice in nurse education. She has also co-edited and published books on study skills. Peggy was awarded a National Teaching Fellowship by the Higher Education Academy in 2014 for her collaborative work on assessment and feedback. Peggy has published and co-presented her work with students nationally and internationally. She currently acts as a co-convenor for the RAISE SIG on partnerships.

Dr Gail Norris (RM, RGN, PhD, MSc, BSc, PG Cert Teaching and Learning Higher Education, senior teaching fellow) is a registered midwife who has spent over 10 years working with pregnant women and their families, and latterly as a team midwife in Forth Valley. Gail began her career in higher education in 2003 at Edinburgh Napier University, and she is now the Lead Midwife for Education. Gail is part of the School's senior leadership team and holds the position of Senior Academic Lead for Student Experience. Gail is a senior teaching fellow and currently teaches both pre-registration and post-registration midwifery students. Her research interests include obesity, particularly during childbirth, completing in 2019 her PhD study *Exploring perception of risk during childbirth in women with a BMI >35kg/m²*.

Jo Pierce qualified as a physiotherapist in 1998 and since this time has worked in numerous acute and primary healthcare settings, specialising in neurological conditions. Her last clinical role was clinical specialist physiotherapist at the Oxford Centre for Enablement (OCE), a tertiary, level 1 centre for the treatment and management of neurological disability. From there she moved into the role of lecturer in physiotherapy and rehabilitation, at Oxford Brookes University, where she is clinical placement lead for the Pre-registration MSc Physiotherapy programme and module lead for the 1st-year neurology content for BSc and Pre-reg MSc. Jo has also taught on the Masters in Rehabilitation course, specifically focusing on the importance of interprofessional working.

Professor Debbie Roberts is Director of the School of Nursing and Allied Health, Liverpool John Moores University. She has deep expertise in nursing, with over 30 years of experience as a qualified nurse, and 20 years as a nurse academic for universities in Wales and England. Debbie's areas of teaching and research expertise include practice and immersive learning, as well as clinical simulation. She has a particular interest in linking research, teaching and innovation; ensuring that evidence-based teaching is used within nurse education and relevant research is embedded into the curriculum. Widely published in the field of nurse education, Prof Roberts has edited a text book (currently being revised as 2nd edition) and contributed to two others used as core texts in nurse education programmes in several countries. She also has published 30 peer-reviewed articles for international journals with her work often cited by others, indicating the impact of her ideas on teaching and learning internationally. Prof Roberts has established a wide range of national and international links through her work as an external examiner and on the editorial board of *Nurse Education in Practice*, and as scientific co-chair of the 2016 NETNEP Global Nurse Education Conference. In 2019, she was nominated as one of the top 100 women in Wales in the inaugural Welsh Women's Awards, which celebrate those women who continue to thrive and excel at the forefront of their professions and make meaningful contributions to the country.

Andrea Surtees (RN, DipHE, BSc Hons, PGCE, MSc) is currently a practice education facilitator (PEF) at Salford Royal Hospital (Salford Care Organisation), which is part of the Northern Care Alliance. She is a nurse by background with 31 years of experience since commencing her training at the Salford School of Nursing in 1989. With the exception of a year living and working as a nurse in Australia she has worked for the same organisation since qualifying in 1992. Her post-registration experiences have taken her across various fields of practice from medicine in the earlier years to surgery later on. During her career she has worked closely with students supporting them initially at ward level both as a mentor and a placement educational lead, then for the past 6 years as a PEF. Andrea is currently the lead for synergy across her care organisation; she has an MSc in Leading Education for Health and Social Care Reform and a keen interest in supporting and developing quality practice learning environments looking at innovative ways to support those who are involved in teaching students in clinical placement, thus helping to cultivate the future workforce of the NHS.

Wendy Sutton works as a matron for paediatrics and neonatal at Mid Cheshire Hospital NHS Foundation Trust. Wendy has over 15 years of experience as a registered paediatric nurse, qualifying from the University of Hertfordshire in 2003 with a Diploma of Higher Education in Child Nursing. Since qualifying, she has undertaken a number of roles within the profession and has successfully completed a BSc (Hons) Enhancing Healthcare Practice and is working towards an MSc Leading Education for Health and Social Care Reform. Wendy began her career at Booth Hall Children's Hospital and has since built a portfolio of experience within children's nursing including specialised surgical care, special education needs, hospice care and nursing education. She has a genuine passion for ensuring all nurses, pre and post registration, receive high-quality learning and she champions high-quality learning environments. Wendy actively supported the development of GM Synergy, a coaching model adopted across Greater Manchester; in 2018, GM Synergy received a Higher Education Academy Collaborative Award for Teaching Excellence and was a finalist in the Student Nursing Times Awards 2019. In her current role she utilises coaching with staff and advocates this approach when supporting others in their practice development.

Zoe Tilley works in physiotherapy education at the University of Nottingham. Her role involves supporting and mentoring students and clinical educators within practice-based learning to ensure quality learning experiences. Previous roles working within clinical practice as a physiotherapist in the fields of trauma, elective orthopaedics and musculoskeletal settings have provided valuable experience of multidisciplinary and interprofessional working. A keen interest in interprofessional working and collaboration has resulted in the development of an online interprofessional programme for healthcare educators and a teaching role on the Foundation to Health Sciences programme within the university. Both programmes have been developed and delivered by a range of healthcare professionals, embedding the philosophy of interprofessional working into the current and future workforce.

FOREWORD

Nursing and midwifery practice along with the provision of nurse and midwife education are in a constant state of flux. The practice of these two professions and the provision of nurse and midwife education are and should always be dynamic entities that adapt and flex to the needs of individuals, families, communities and nations. The Nursing and Midwifery Council has introduced a number of new standards that detail the skills and knowledge that will be required of the next generation of nurses and midwives to enable them to deliver care that is patient focused, safe and effective. *Supervising and Assessing Student Nurses and Midwives in Clinical Practice: a practical guide* is timely; this is the go-to book to help practitioners and students get the most out of practice learning, aligned to the professional regulator's standards.

With change there is often a sense of uncertainty, a raft of questions and queries that need answers. Roberts and Leigh's *Supervising and Assessing Student Nurses and Midwives in Clinical Practice* provides the answers that will enable all of those nurses and midwives who have or will have an active role in supervising and assessing student nurses and midwives in the practice setting to understand and apply the principles of practice learning, wherever this may occur.

Supervising and Assessing Student Nurses and Midwives in Clinical Practice has been written by professionals in the field who are well versed in teaching and learning from a wide range of perspectives. This is a contemporary text that is truly a practical guide that steers and supports. It is written in an accessible and user-friendly way, helping the reader see through the complexities that are inherently associated with practice assessment.

I was delighted to have been asked to write this foreword; teaching and learning in practice are activities that are very close to my heart and I know close to the hearts of other nurses and midwives. I sincerely recommend this book to students and practitioners who learn and practise together with the overall goal of offering high-quality care that is safe and effective.

Professor Ian Peate
OBE FRCN

ABBREVIATIONS

AHP	Allied health professional
ANTT	Aseptic non-touch technique
CAIPE	Centre for the Advancement of Interprofessional Education
CFT	Compassion-focused therapy
CMT	Compassionate mind training
CPR	Cardiopulmonary resuscitation
DNAR	Do not attempt resuscitation
GMC	General Medical Council
GP	General practitioner
HCPC	Health and Care Professions Council
HEI	Higher education institution
ICU	Intensive care unit
IDT/MDT	Interdisciplinary / multidisciplinary team: these terms have been used to describe the wider team involved in patient care to include health care workers, therapy assistants, family members and volunteers as examples
IP	Interprofessional
IPE	Interprofessional education
IPL	Interprofessional learning
ISTEL	Integrated simulation and technology enhanced learning
LO	Learning outcome
NMC	Nursing and Midwifery Council
OSCE	Objective structured clinical examination
OT	Occupational therapy / therapist
PDA	Pre, during and after
RCOG	Royal College of Obstetricians and Gynaecologists

SBE	Simulation-based education
SLT	Speech and language therapy / therapist
SNT	Staff nurse toolkit
SP	Simulated patient
SRB	Soothing rhythm breathing
SWOT	Strengths, weaknesses, opportunities, threats
VCSE	Voluntary, community and social enterprise
VR	Virtual reality
WHO	World Health Organization

INTRODUCTION

This book is written at an important time in nurse education in the UK. The professional nursing and midwifery body in the UK (Nursing and Midwifery Council, NMC) undertook a 2-year consultation with a range of key stakeholder groups such as students, educators, healthcare professionals, charities and patient groups from across the UK. *Future nurse: Standards of proficiency for registered nurses* was published in 2018 (NMC, 2018a). The NMC refers to the standards as:

> *"ambitious new standards that set out the skills and knowledge the next generation of nurses will learn to enable them to deliver world class care".* (NMC, 2018b)

At the same time, the NMC published *Realising Professionalism: Standards for education and training* (NMC, 2018c), which are set out in three parts:

Part 1 *Standards framework for nursing and midwifery education.* This document provides a framework of five headings that underpin nurse education and training:
1. Learning culture
2. Educational governance and quality
3. Student learning and empowerment
4. Educators and assessors
5. Curricula and assessment.

Part 2 *Standards for student supervision and assessment.* This document sets out the expectations for the learning, support, supervision and assessment (of theory and practice) of students in the practice environment. It includes two important annexe sections outlining specific proficiencies which must be achieved by the end of the programme.

Part 3 *Programme standards, the standards specific for each pre-registration or post-registration programme.* This document sets out the legal requirements for all pre-registration nursing education programmes.

Collectively the four documents contain proficiencies that specify the knowledge and skills that registered nurses must demonstrate when caring for people of all ages and across all care settings, reflecting what the public can expect nurses to know and be able to do in order to deliver safe, compassionate and effective nursing care (Leigh and Roberts, 2018). The new NMC *Future nurse: Standards of proficiency for registered nurses* can be accessed here: www.nmc.org.uk/globalassets/sitedocuments/education-standards/future-nurse-proficiencies.pdf

PRACTICE SUPERVISORS AND PRACTICE ASSESSORS

The NMC (2018c) standards *Part 2: Standards for student supervision and assessment* outline new roles to support learning and assessment in clinical practice. These new standards include a shift away from the role of mentor (who previously undertook both teaching and assessor roles), to two new separate roles of **practice supervisor** and **practice assessor** and a new role of **academic assessor**. Part two of the NMC standards can be accessed here: www.nmc.org.uk/globalassets/sitedocuments/education-standards/student-supervision-assessment.pdf

Leigh and Roberts (2018) provide an outline of the roles and responsibilities in *Boxes 1–3*:

Box 1: Summary of role and responsibilities for the practice supervisor

Serve as role models for safe and effective practice in line with their code of conduct
Support learning in line with their scope of practice to enable the student to meet their proficiencies and programme outcomes
Support and supervise students, providing feedback on their progress towards, and achievement of, proficiencies and skills
Receive ongoing support to participate in the practice learning of students

Box 2: Summary of role and responsibilities for the practice assessor

Conduct assessments to confirm student achievement of proficiencies and programme outcomes for practice learning
Make assessment decisions that are informed by feedback sought and received from practice supervisors

Box 2: *(cont'd)*

Make and record objective, evidence-based assessments on conduct, proficiency and achievement, drawing on student records, direct observations, student self-reflection and other resources
Work in partnership with the nominated academic assessor to evaluate and recommend the student for progression for each part of the programme, in line with programme standards and local and national policies
Provide sufficient opportunities for the practice assessor to periodically observe the student across environments in order to inform decisions for assessment and progression

Box 3: *Summary of role and responsibilities for the academic assessor*

Collate and confirm student achievement of proficiencies and programme outcomes in the academic environment for each part of the programme; making and recording objective, evidence-based decisions and recommendations for progression, drawing on student records and other resources
Have an understanding of the student's learning and achievement in practice
Work in partnership with a nominated practice assessor to evaluate and recommend the student for progression for each part of the programme
Communication and collaboration between academic and practice assessors is scheduled for relevant points in programme structure and student progression

It should be remembered that each higher education institution (HEI) in partnership with placement providers may have different arrangements for operationalising these roles; so how each role appears where you are based may be slightly different, although the principles are all the same.

WHO IS THIS BOOK FOR?

The book is aimed at all those nurses and midwives who have or will have an active role in supervising and assessing student nurses and midwives in the practice setting. In addition, for the first time individuals from disciplines other than nursing and midwifery are also now able to supervise learning, and therefore allied health professional (AHP) colleagues might also want to refer to the book for hints and tips on supporting student learning. The new NMC educational standards also require all new registrants to be 'supervisor ready' and therefore the book might also be useful for final-year students who are aspiring to take on the supervisor role at the point of qualification.

Outcome 5.8 (NMC, 2018a) states the requirement to support and supervise students in the delivery of nursing care, promoting reflection and providing constructive feedback, and evaluating and documenting their performance.

The role of the practice assessor is also new (and has been separated from that of the supervisor), indicating the importance of objective and thorough assessment of learning in clinical practice. Different health boards and NHS Trusts (together with HEIs) will make potentially different decisions about who undertakes the practice assessor role, but the principles of assessment will remain constant, and it is those principles that this book will focus on.

This book seeks to help those supporting students to learn in clinical practice to understand and apply the principles of practice learning. Nurse education programmes tend to introduce information and gradually build on concepts and ideas as the student progresses through the programme (Pront and McNeill, 2019). Although lessons learned in the classroom are important, it is in the clinical practice arena where students learn to recognise and apply theoretical knowledge in the real world. The book has been designed to be a practical resource; a straightforward 'how to' guide for anyone supporting or assessing learning in clinical practice. Each chapter is underpinned by contemporary evidence related to clinical learning and assessment. Each author or group of authors draws on a wide range of contemporary global evidence and applies this to a UK context. There are exercises for the reader to complete to promote thinking and consideration of how to bring the ideas to life across a range of clinical settings.

STRUCTURE OF THE BOOK

The book is laid out in a series of chapters that each addresses a different aspect of supervision and assessment in and through clinical practice. The book is designed to be used as a practical guide, and as such you may wish to read it from beginning to end, or dip in and out of various chapters as they become useful to you. There are activities to do in each chapter which will help you to frame the issues in relation to yourself and/or your team where you work. Some chapters also include scenarios based on typical real-life situations which you can use to apply the principles outlined in the book, or which will help you to see how the standards and the learning associated with the standards can be used in supervision and assessment. Each clinical area is different and so the book aims to help you to consider areas outside your own sphere of practice in order to prepare for supervision and assessment in your particular context. The authors of this book understand that in the real world of clinical practice, learning opportunities can present themselves at any time in an *ad hoc* and disorganised fashion. This book is designed to help you to plan for the learning opportunities that it is possible to plan for, to consider what is possible for learning and assessment in your area, and to get ready for and deliver the best learning experiences that you can for the learners in order to prepare them for their role as future nurses.

Chapter 1 focuses on the clinical learning environment and the context of learning and assessment. The activities in this chapter are important because you will be asked to return to your responses to these activities elsewhere in the book.

Chapter 2 explores the culture for practice learning through developing the education team. Concepts of leadership are explored and used to set the scene for effective approaches to supervision and assessment. The education team will of course include the three new roles outlined by the NMC: supervisor, assessor and academic assessor, but it has long been recognised that students learn from everyone that they come into contact with in the clinical learning environment. This chapter therefore discusses the importance of building a culture where learning and practice development is everyone's business.

Chapter 3 will introduce the reader to coaching models such as Clinical Learning in Practice (CLiP) and GM Synergy with their embedded core coaching concepts. These include use of effective listening and questioning skills to facilitate learning. The focus here is on developing the skills to engage in coaching conversations, developing the coach–student expectations and promoting wellbeing.

Chapter 4 covers interprofessional supervision of student learning and provides an overview of the approaches to learning that are common across disciplines and discusses the opportunities for interprofessional learning in practice. While students have always learned from a range of individuals within the clinical learning area, the new NMC educational standards have formalised the role of interprofessional supervision of student learning, enabling all those who are active on a professional register to support student nurses and midwives with their learning. Through interactions with a variety of providers, students learn about the roles of other disciplines and how to collaborate in a team. Although it is acknowledged that each profession will have a distinct and unique skills set, individuals can still teach students from other professions.

Chapter 5 provides practical guidance on providing students with feedback on their clinical practice. The chapter outlines a range of strategies to ensure that feedback is provided in an honest, open and positive manner using feedforward techniques that enable and support student development. The chapter also includes ideas about how to manage difficult conversations to support students who may be struggling with a range of elements associated with clinical learning such as practical skills development, psychomotor skills, communication and assertiveness and/or linking theory to practice.

Chapter 6 looks at challenging situations and principled decision-making in the supervisory and assessment relationship through a midwifery lens. This chapter explores strategies for building resilience in the workforce through empowering assessors, supervisors and students to develop their own leadership skills and through introducing restorative practices. You will be introduced to self-soothing exercises creating affiliative feelings for our own struggles which can help when making the difficult assessment and supervisory decisions. The chapter will also outline a range of approaches to enable difficult and challenging conversations to take place. The chapter can be used by both midwives and nurses in clinical supervision and assessor roles.

Chapter 7 provides an overview of the nature of clinical assessment and what it means to be proficient. The skills of assessment are outlined together with some exercises to encourage readers to develop their questioning and assessment skills. The chapter discusses how practice assessors will cope with students on different programmes at varying academic levels; for example: students that already have a degree in and may be undertaking a master's level pre-registration nursing programme. A range of approaches to assessment are discussed in relation to the NMC requirement for practice assessors to link with academic assessors. The role of patients or service users in assessment will also be discussed.

Chapter 8 covers the use of simulation-based education for supervision and assessment of student learning. This chapter will provide an overview of the range of healthcare simulation and discuss the benefits of enabling students to learn in safe, supportive, simulated environments. The chapter outlines how simulation-based education (SBE) can be integrated into nursing and midwifery education as a useful adjunct to the real world of clinical practice to support student learning. The chapter will encourage readers to think about how they might use various SBE approaches and techniques in order to achieve the NMC proficiencies, while also refining holistic or person-centred nursing or midwifery skills. The new NMC standards ask new registrants to be 'supervisor' ready. The role of SBE to support learners to fulfil the requirements of practice supervisors at the point of registration will also be discussed.

Chapter 9 explores the future of practice learning, applying the core concepts of a learning organisation to promote excellence (quality and governance); it therefore looks at the whole picture, considering strategies that enable creative thinking around innovative student learning experiences. Explored is the application of leadership knowledge and skills that when used effectively create the right environment whereby practice learning can flourish. Activities in this chapter include being introduced to a scenario about setting up a community of practice, providing opportunities to reflect, plan and develop strategies to sustain clinical practice as an effective and key environment where student learning can take place.

We hope that you will use the book regularly, engaging with the range of activities and scenarios presented to you that will help you to support students in achieving proficiency against the new NMC (2018a) standards. The activities are designed to be practical in nature and will help you to apply the principles described in each chapter to your own work context. The scenarios outline real-life examples that demonstrate the principles in action and again can be adapted to where you work. If you are a student nurse, this book might help you to think about your role as a Future Practice supervisor, and Future Nurse.

REFERENCES

Leigh, J. and Roberts, D. (2018) Critical exploration of the new NMC standards of proficiency for registered nurses. *British Journal of Nursing*, **27(18)**: 1068–72.

Nursing and Midwifery Council (2018a) *Future nurse: standards of proficiency for registered nurses*. NMC. Available at www.nmc.org. uk/globalassets/sitedocuments/education-standards/future-nurse-proficiencies.pdf (accessed 13 August 2020).

Nursing and Midwifery Council (2018b) *New NMC standards shape the future of nursing for next generation*. NMC. Available at www.nmc. org.uk/news/press-releases/new-nmc-standards-shape-the-future-of-nursing-for-next-generation (accessed 13 August 2020).

Nursing and Midwifery Council (2018c) *Realising Professionalism: Standards for education and training*. NMC. Available at www.nmc. org.uk/standards/standards-for-nurses (accessed 15 January 2021).

Pront, L. and McNeill, L. (2019) Nursing students' perceptions of a clinical learning assessment activity: 'Linking the puzzle pieces of theory to practice'. *Nurse Education in Practice*, **36:** 85–90. doi: 10.1016/j. nepr.2019.03.008

CHAPTER 1

THE CONTEXT OF PRACTICE SUPERVISION AND ASSESSMENT

Debbie Roberts

1.1 INTRODUCTION

This chapter outlines the context of practice supervision and assessment; and emphasises the importance of the clinical context or environment where learning and assessment take place. This is important for two reasons: firstly, nurses (and others) are expected to help the students to make links between different service delivery and practice locations; so for example, practice supervisors may see students who have had a vast variety of previous clinical experience in a range of settings and who will need help to compare and contrast approaches to care delivery. Secondly, practice supervisors may support students from any field of nursing practice. Previously, mentors and students were expected to be from the same field of nursing practice (this was known as 'due regard'), but this requirement no longer exists, meaning that nurses who are experienced within an area of clinical practice can support student learning (and assessment) regardless of which field of practice the student is from. It will be important, therefore, for practice supervisors and assessors to be able to help the students to consider how their clinical learning could be applied to their own relevant field of practice or in different practice contexts.

We will explain how nurses (and others) responsible for supporting or supervising student learning can use the approaches described across a range of contexts, fields of practice and geographical boundaries. The book will therefore apply to all fields of practice (and midwifery) and clinical contexts. Learning and teaching in clinical practice are heavily influenced by context; and furthermore, the context of care is changing over time (Jack and Hamshire, 2019).

It is perhaps important to acknowledge that supervising and assessing student nurses is not the only role for practice supervisors and assessors; rather the role is in addition to, and often secondary to, delivering patient care. Reynolds *et al.* (2020) make the important point that learning and care delivery should not be seen as two separate things. Indeed, they argue very strongly for practice supervisors and assessors to not only see themselves as educators, but to align learning with care delivery. They discuss what they refer to as the creation of teachable moments; a concept which we endorse and which is returned to throughout the book.

After reading this chapter you will be able to:

- Identify and consider the learning opportunities that are common within your clinical area, and those which are unique to your setting
- Begin to think about the knowledge and skills that learners may have acquired elsewhere and how these might be applied or further developed under your supervision in your area
- Begin to think about how you might support learners from all fields of nursing practice or who are from other disciplines.

1.2 CLINICAL WISDOM

For many years (since the 1990s) learning to be a nurse or midwife in the UK has been equally divided between classroom and practical or clinical placement experience. The NMC *Emergency standards for nursing and midwifery education* (NMC, 2020) introduced during the COVID-19 pandemic briefly removed this requirement. These emergency standards however were temporary, aimed purely as a response to the unprecedented situation of the pandemic. Students are supported and guided through clinical placements by registered nurses/midwives, who take on the major responsibility for student learning and assessment in practice settings. Registrants are expected to pass on their clinical or professional wisdom to students. Effective clinical learning involves registered nurses/midwives and others who are able to be effective role models and who have an ability to pass on their craft knowledge or professional wisdom.

McKie *et al.* (2012) explain wisdom in three formulations: philosophical, religious and psychological. The philosophical draws on classical ancient Greek ideas on wisdom as a virtue. Religions seek to instil wisdom in followers so that they may recognise the existence of the divine creator. People seek answers and practical guidance in order to live well as a result. The psychological outlines the science of human strengths, which includes reflective thinking. They go on to say that clinical wisdom is a feature of reflective judgement, and being able to practise within local and particular contexts; and they further suggest that clinical wisdom can be acquired, maintained and fostered through reflection.

✍ ACTIVITY 1.1

Start to think about your clinical wisdom and whether or how you see yourself as an educator.
This is a personal reflective activity, so no answer guide is provided.

In order to gain such clinical wisdom, students spend time on clinical practice placements where they experience emotional and cognitive engagement in order to address the complex, fast paced and sometimes uncertain nature of care (McKie *et al.*, 2012). Indeed, Lord Willis (2015) in his influential report *Shape of caring: A review of the future education and training of registered nurses and care assistants* discusses how nurses will be required to possess advanced knowledge and skills in the future. The report considers the future of nurse education and preparation in light of recognised care failings. The report says:

> "*Nurses must be educated to deliver excellent standards of evidence-based clinical care themselves; they must think critically in order to make decisions and provide judgement while also delegating fundamental aspects of care to others who are sufficiently trained and who operate under their supervision*". (Willis, 2015, p. 14)

You can access the full report here:
www.hee.nhs.uk/sites/default/files/documents/2348-Shape-of-caring-review-FINAL.pdf

The report by Willis (2015) was one of the influential pieces of work that guided the development of the NMC *Future nurse: Standards of proficiency for registered nurses* (NMC, 2018).

Learning in clinical practice must be guided by mastering principles of practice. Pront and McNeill (2019) suggest that:

> "*In health education, this is confounded by the fact that no two patients are the same, presentations for the same disease can vary and each patient interaction is unique. Consequently, nursing education focuses on the principles of practice aimed at building transferable knowledge for application to any setting or situation*".

It is the role of the **practice supervisor** to encourage and educate the student to apply the principles of nursing; to recognise important cues; relate these to theoretical concepts and to act, using evidence-based interventions. McClure and Black (2013) discuss the importance of the **clinical preceptor** (an American term for someone that supports student learning in clinical practice) through an integrative literature review. The authors describe the instrumental nature of clinical learning and the role of the preceptor as complex and multifaceted.

Jack and Hamshire (2019) suggest an interactive Practice Learning and Teaching Orientations Tool (PLATO), which builds on four personal orientations:

- **Role model** This includes personal thoughts about how you act as a role model and asks the individual to think about identification of role modelling opportunities and how role modelling practice could be analysed
- **Advocate** Being familiar with the learner's needs, supporting learners to access appropriate learning opportunities and trying to identify the most important thing that influences self as student advocate
- **Legitimiser** Developing a positive mindset in self and valuing the qualities of the learner
- **Respecter** Finding ways to seek out the qualities and strengths of learners; considering personal views about the learner's stage of development and ensuring active, meaningful participation.

The tool is offered as a means to help educators in the clinical setting to support their students and also to support personal development. The tool focuses on identifying personal strengths in self and others; as such it is offered as an affirmative "process of positive change, inspiring positive possibilities with a collective forward-thinking vision, uncovering and bringing forth existing strengths" (Jack and Hamshire, 2019).

☑ ACTIVITY 1.2

Download the paper by Jack and Hamshire (2019) and look at Figure 2:
- Try to answer the various prompt questions yourself and then perhaps ask fellow supervisors and assessors to join you in a wider discussion of their responses.
- Think about how you will bring the four educator orientations to life.

This is a personal reflective activity, so no answer guide is provided.

✎ ACTIVITY 1.3

Access the NMC (2018) *Future nurse: Standards of proficiency for registered nurses* and highlight all those outcome statements that could apply to the examples in this chapter. Start to think about how as a practice supervisor you will link some of the outcome statements together and help students to apply them to different populations and contexts of care.

Think about students at different stages of the programme: you can repeat this exercise and begin to make increasingly complex links between the various outcome statements and proficiencies. What will you be looking for in a student in the first, second or third years of a programme? What will you expect the student to demonstrate at each stage of the programme?

An answer guide is provided at the end of this chapter.

✎ ACTIVITY 1.4

If you are a clinical supervisor, you should develop a table of the learning opportunities that are open to students (from all fields of nursing practice) within your area. You can then discuss with practice assessors how these activities can be used as part of the assessment process against the NMC (2018) *Future nurse: Standards of proficiency for registered nurses*. The learning opportunities can also be used as a springboard for discussion and reflection on practice between practice supervisor and student (Perrin and Scott, 2016).

An answer guide is provided at the end of this chapter.

1.3 THE CHANGING LANDSCAPE

The landscape of nursing and midwifery has changed over recent decades; nursing care is delivered in a wider range of contexts than ever before. Inpatient hospital stays are shorter than ever and people are nursed in community settings with much higher acuity than ever before. Nursing services span urban and rural settings, with an increasing emphasis on providing care that is closer to home (Zwakhalen *et al.*, 2018).

There are several NMC (2018) outcome statements that could be applied to the situations outlined in this chapter that newly qualified nurses from any field of nursing practice should demonstrate at the point of registration. We will now consider some specific contexts in which clinical learning can take place and suggest ways in which this can be facilitated and supported by supervisors. As a practice supervisor, you may work in a single setting, but it might be useful to consider other clinical settings that the student has experienced or will experience later in the programme, so that you can help the student to draw comparisons or prepare for future placements. Ion *et al.* (2020) explain this in the following way from a mental health nursing perspective; they say: "a broad assessment of a nursing student's interpersonal skills is not the same as a focused assessment of their ability to provide support for someone who, for example, has revealed a history of domestic violence or sexual abuse". So, as a practice supervisor or as part of a team of supervisors, you will need to think about what you are looking for in your particular context for each of the standards.

Students often require practice supervisors to flag-up or make learning opportunities explicit during care delivery, rather than seeing the learning as something that happens when there is nothing else left to do. Teachable moments (as defined by Reynolds *et al.*, 2020) can be identified in partnership with patients and carers in order to help students to explore key points in care delivery and of the experience of those receiving care. They go on to point out that this requires a team approach to create a safe space for open communication and reflection to take place. Even though nursing care delivery is often fast paced and taking place with a level of uncertainty, it is possible to integrate learning opportunities into the structure of the day; examples cited by Reynolds *et al.* (2020) include:

> "*Learning may be included as standard on routine meeting agendas and identifying learning opportunities can be incorporated into the structure of huddles in the clinical setting for the benefit of the team as well as learners. In this way, potential T-moments can be harnessed, and learning embedded more fully within a team or organisation*".

But in order to do this, it is important that practice supervisors and assessors (as individuals and teams) think about, and get ready for, the range of learning opportunities that are available to learners.

1.3.1 Community placements

The Willis (2015) report suggests that community placements will take on an increasingly important significance as numerous learning opportunities are available to support the development of student nurses in community settings. The report emphasises a shift in the context of care, and one which nurse education should mirror. Community placements can help student nurses to begin to understand how experiences and environmental factors can influence health and illness across the lifespan. The link between the environment and health (and subsequent influences on ill health) features heavily in the new NMC educational standards (NMC, 2018). Perrin and Scott (2016) provide a useful overview of the contribution of **health visitors** to the pre-registration education of student nurses in the children and young people field; the paper includes a table (p. 46) of 32 typical learning opportunities, including, for example:

- Interprofessional working
- Engaging with baby-friendly initiative
- Child development, milestones and deviations
- Community profiling
- Chairing and minuting team, professional and core group meetings
- Family planning
- Using health promotion and health education models
- Immunisations and vaccinations
- Writing reports, letters and minute-taking skill
- Non-medical prescribing opportunities.

Try to obtain the paper from the reference list. The paper by Perrin and Scott (2016) also highlights an example of the student's experience within a health visitor placement (see Box 1, Perrin and Scott, 2016). From the description it is possible to see the influence of the placement and how the student has been nurtured by the health visitor. The description from the student nurse also demonstrates how links from one context of care can be applied elsewhere.

1.3.2 Care of older people

Across the UK there are increasing numbers of older people living at home with a wide range of chronic illnesses; and there is an increasing emphasis on trying to ensure that older people can remain independent and live at home (Department of Health, 2014). There is some tentative evidence that students see nursing in community settings as unappealing because of the chronic disease profile and high workload (van Iersel *et al.*, 2016).

In a study conducted in the USA in which reflective diaries of students working with people with long-term conditions in community settings were analysed, the findings revealed that they were able to learn:

> *"about three main aspects of living with chronic conditions: beliefs about chronic conditions, managing chronic conditions, and experiencing chronic conditions".* (Olson *et al.*, 2018)

The study found that the writing of reflective diaries (which the authors refer to as journaling) revealed how the students had developed learning partnerships with the older people which helped them to understand the experience of living with a chronic condition as an older adult. Importantly, the students also began to appreciate the highly skilled nature of working with older people with chronic conditions (Olson *et al.*, 2018). Interestingly, collaboration is evident on a number of different levels, including between researchers and students. The study highlights the importance and centrality of relationships to nursing care and to student learning.

✏ ACTIVITY 1.5

As a practice supervisor, how will you help student nurses from all four fields of practice gain valuable, positive learning experiences when working with people with long-term conditions where you work? How does your setting (or context) impact on the care that you provide, and how can you help the student to gain an understanding of these issues?

This is a personal reflective activity, so no answer guide is provided.

1.3.3 Health promotion

The new NMC (2018) *Future nurse: Standards of proficiency for registered nurses* contains a whole platform relating to promoting health and preventing ill health: "standard 2.10 provides information in accessible ways to help people understand and make decisions about their health, life choices, illness and care".

✏ ACTIVITY 1.6

Start to consider how the new standards ask nurses from all four fields of nursing practice to implement Standard 2.10, and how to provide accessible information. For example, if your patient has a learning disability, then accessibility to information might include visual or easy read information; if the patient has a sensory disability such as sight and/or hearing loss, how is information made accessible to them?

An answer guide is provided at the end of this chapter.

It is possible for nurses to engage in health-promotion activities within urgent treatment centres. Nurses can use opportunistic brief health-promotion intervention to help people to understand modifiable risk factors (Chacha-Mannie *et al.*, 2020):

> "*Brief health promotion interventions are structured ways of providing advice to people, using methods such as motivational*

interviewing and opportunistic contact to raise awareness, assess readiness to engage and prompt behaviour change. They are based on motivational interviewing techniques, which involve a non-confrontational and non-judgmental approach".

Motivational interview techniques are highlighted by the NMC as an evidence-based best practice communication skill required by newly qualified nurses at the point of registration (NMC, 2018).

1.3.4 Rural healthcare

Rural healthcare is becoming increasingly important. Typically, rural areas have a population density of fewer than 150 persons per square kilometre but definitions of rurality are varied; for example, in the UK, the Office for National Statistics (2011) refers to populations of less than 10 000 as being rural and those with a population of above 10 000 as being urban. What is clear, however, is that access to health services can be challenging in rural areas, and health beliefs and values may be different to urban areas; as a result, there may be differences in health-seeking behaviours (Roberts *et al.*, 2014). The role of the nurse may subsequently be very different.

Internationally, there is evidence that nurses have adapted their role to meet rural patients' needs, but the scale of rurality is often accentuated. For example, Hounsgaard *et al.* (2013) describe the issues facing nurses in rural Greenland and highlight the importance of being able to undertake a range of non-clinical tasks such as shovelling snow and applying salt-grit to pavements, distributing post and being an all-round community worker. Hounsgaard *et al.* (2013) demonstrate the difficulties encountered for the nurses serving the remote and rural areas of Greenland in separating social work from health-related issues, and argue that nurses adapt their role to meet patient needs. In some areas of the UK, new roles are emerging to support patient needs in other ways. For example, the Scottish Family Nurse Partnership prepares nurses to support first-time mothers in rural Scotland during pregnancy through to the child's second birthday. The role focuses on preventative health practices with the following three aims:

- to improve pregnancy and birth outcomes, through improved prenatal health behaviours
- to improve child health and development, through positive, responsive caregiving, and
- to improve the economic self-sufficiency of the family, through developing a vision and plans for the future.

In Wales, there is evidence that taking mobile health surgeries out to farmers enables on-the-spot blood pressure testing and opportunities for discussion on mental health and wellbeing (Davies *et al.*, 2019). Furthermore, Davies *et al.* describe how farmers can become isolated with limited opportunities for wider social interaction, which in turn can impinge on mental health. This is compounded when farmers can feel that being in a small rural community makes them hesitant to use wellbeing services for fear of breaches in confidentiality and privacy. Because of this, peer-to-peer wellbeing services are being developed to support farmers in rural Wales. The report also discusses the importance of designing services in cooperation with those who will use the services. While the report is specifically discussing a project aimed at farmers, this approach could be applied to other socially isolated groups; so there may be similar examples that you could draw on to direct the student to in your locality.

ACTIVITY 1.7

Think about the nursing roles in rural communities and how nurses can be pivotal in enhancing the wellbeing of remote and hard-to-reach communities. You might also begin to think about the overlap between health and social care provision. You may not work in a rural community, but there may still be 'hard-to-reach groups'. Think about who these groups might be where you work; and devise ways in which you can help students to be aware of them.

An answer guide is provided at the end of this chapter.

For further information you might like to read Adamson *et al.* (2016) (see *Recommended further reading* for the full reference). The paper discusses the changing nature of day hospitals and their role in modern healthcare, and highlights the importance of person-centred care.

1.3.5 Urban healthcare

Most people in the UK live in urban areas. *Future nurse: Standards of proficiency for registered nurses* (NMC, 2018) acknowledges the changes in society and has prepared the new standards in order for future nurses to be able to care for people across all settings "empowering people, communities and populations to exercise choice, take control of their own health decisions and behaviours, and by supporting people to manage their own care where possible". As a practice supervisor, it is crucial that you are able to consider the full range of care settings and populations that students will need to be conversant with in order for them to meet the relevant NMC standards. The students should be prepared to engage with different populations in order to fulfil their role against the seven NMC (2018) platforms.

The *Five year forward view* and the follow-up report *Next steps on the NHS five year forward view* (NHS England 2014, 2017) call for better integration of health and care with better locally led community care. Care delivery, therefore, is being moved closer to home; students are very likely to require more placement time in these areas where care is delivered closer to home, or in placements where new ways of working are being implemented. As a practice supervisor it will be important for you to be aware of such developments in your area so that you can plan learning opportunities for students. Increasingly, there is a recognition that there is a link between the environment and public health. Healthy living should be a part of everyone's life. New partnerships are developing across England between housing development demonstrator sites to explore new models of healthcare delivery. For further information see Bowkett and Norman (2018) from *Recommended further reading*. Housing conditions across the UK vary significantly, and housing is a social determinant of health. You might want to download the World Health Organization (WHO) recommendations:

WHO *Housing and health guidelines* (2018): https://apps.who.int/iris/bitstream/handle/10665/276001/9789241550376-eng.pdf?ua=1

The WHO (2018) report makes some recommendations concerning housing to support health and wellbeing. There is emerging evidence that providing social support for older adults in urban settings results in improved health and wellbeing outcomes, and reduced health service costs (Warwick-Booth *et al.*, 2019). The pilot project carried out in England by Warwick-Booth *et al.* describes the development of what they term an 'age friendly community' providing holistic support for older people. If projects like this are being developed where you work, as a practice assessor or supervisor you could try to ensure that these developments are communicated to your higher education institution (HEI) team and incorporated into nurse education programmes.

At the other end of the lifespan, there is also evidence that adolescents, particularly girls (aged 15–19), are disproportionately high users of emergency services at two centres in London (Gnani *et al.*, 2014). In that study undertaken at two co-located general practitioner (GP)-led urgent care centres in London, adolescents were more likely to attend the centres than routine general practice. Many of those attending were seeking advice for conditions often seen in primary care settings such as musculoskeletal conditions and injuries and respiratory tract infections (Gnani *et al.*, 2014). In the UK, GP-led urgent care centres were initially developed to reduce accident and emergency attendances and resultant short-stay hospital admissions. The paper outlines the centres and the model of care provided. Often this population group is considered to be 'healthy' with minimal need; however, the respondents in the study wanted to speak to a healthcare professional about sex, sexually transmitted diseases, contraception and pregnancy, acne, smoking, diet, exercise, weight and nutrition (Gnani *et al.*, 2014). These are areas where nurses have a duty of care to promote health and prevent ill health: platform 2 of the NMC (2018) *Future nurse: Standards of proficiency for registered nurses.*

ACTIVITY 1.8

Think about how the role of the nurse in promoting health and preventing ill health might be different in an urban setting compared with a community setting. If you are a practice supervisor working in an emergency centre and an adolescent woman attends for a wrist injury, how can you use this example as a learning opportunity?

An answer guide is provided at the end of this chapter.

TOP TIP

There may be similar centres within the placement circuit where you are working; if so, as a practice supervisor, you may want to see if there are opportunities to offer placements in this area. This may require some support from the HEI, but could be a valuable learning opportunity for students.

Just as there are hard-to-reach communities in rural areas, this phenomenon is also evident in urban areas. It is well known that the homeless population often have complex health needs; many are not registered with a GP and therefore access to healthcare is poor. Elwell-Sutton *et al.* (2016) describe what they term as a tri-morbidity of a combination of physical illness, mental illness and substance misuse affecting this population; furthermore, they point out that homelessness exists in many forms. The study shows that "access to primary care appears to be influenced by the type of homelessness which people are experiencing, with rough sleepers having the worst access and lowest rates of utilization". The Mental Health Foundation (2013) points out that both physical and mental health have common factors and are not fundamentally different. The report calls for a closer integration of mental and physical health services; as a result, there may be emerging roles for nurses.

 TOP TIP

If you are a practice supervisor, try to develop a network of opportunities where new and emerging roles are being established and enquire if such areas might be open to taking students. This might require some negotiating with the HEI to develop other practice supervisors.

The impact for students in undertaking a placement with hard-to-reach populations is demonstrated by an interesting study conducted with nursing students in the USA by Garner and Emory (2018). The study suggests that interacting with vulnerable populations (such as the homeless) enables students to gain valuable insights into the particular health challenges and experiences of these populations. Furthermore, in doing so, students are enabled to reframe their own (often preconceived) ideas: decreasing their fear, increasing their empathy and enhancing their understanding of the role of the nurse as advocate (Garner and Emory, 2018). At the point of registration newly qualified nurses must be able to demonstrate proficiency in:

> *"1.14 Provide and promote non-discriminatory, person-centred and sensitive care at all times, reflecting on people's values and beliefs, diverse backgrounds, cultural characteristics, language requirements, needs and preferences, taking account of any need for adjustments"*
>
> *"3.4 Understand and apply a person-centred approach to nursing care, demonstrating shared assessment, planning, decision making and goal setting when working with people, their families, communities and populations of all ages".*
> (NMC, 2018)

1.4 SUMMARY

This chapter highlights the changing nature and context of nursing; with an increasing emphasis on providing care closer to home. The chapter positions learning and teaching as something which should be integrated with care delivery, rather than seen as a separate entity. The chapter has highlighted some specific issues in rural and urban communities and asked practice-based teams and supervisors to begin to identify the range of learning opportunities that are available, and the application of the NMC (2018) outcome statements to their specific area of practice. It has long been known that learning in clinical practice is valued by students; and that the staff who work alongside students act as inspirational role models. The chapter calls for all nurses to see themselves as educators and to include teaching within their everyday work with patients and clients.

RECOMMENDED FURTHER READING

Adamson, E., Pow, J., Houston, F. and Redpath, P. (2016) Exploring the experiences of patients attending day hospitals in rural Scotland: capturing the patient's voice. *Journal of Clinical Nursing*, **26(19–20):** 3044–55. doi: 10.1111/jocn.13651

Bowkett, A. and Norman, H. (2018) NHS Healthy New Towns Programme. *Planning Theory and Practice*, **19(4):** 628–32. doi: 10.1080/14649357.2018.1435245

Health Education England. *Bitesized teaching.* Available at: www. hee.nhs.uk/our-work/mental-health/bitesized-teaching (accessed 13 August 2020).

World Health Organization (2020) *State of the world's nursing 2020.* Geneva: WHO. Available at: https://apps.who.int/iris/rest/ bitstreams/1274201/retrieve (accessed 13 August 2020).

REFERENCES

Chacha-Mannie, C., Pallikadavath, S., Dewy, A. *et al.* (2020) Exploring the effectiveness of a brief health promotion intervention in an urgent treatment centre. *Primary Health Care,* **30(2):** 27–33. doi: 10.7748/ phc.2020.e1608

Davies, A.R., Homolova, L., Grey, C.N.B., Fisher, J., Burchett, N. and Kousoulis, A. (2019) *Supporting farming communities at times of uncertainty: An action framework to support the mental health and well-being of farmers and their families.* Public Health Wales NHS Trust and Mental Health Foundation.

Department of Health (2014) *Transforming primary care.* Department of Health.

Elwell-Sutton, T., Fok, J., Albanese, F., Mathie, H. and Holland, R. (2016) Factors associated with access to care and healthcare utilization in the homeless population of England. *Journal of Public Health,* **39(1):** 26–33. doi:10.1093/pubmed/fdw008

Garner, J. and Emory, J. (2018) Changing students' perceptions of the homeless: A community service learning experience. *Nurse Education in Practice*, **29**: 133–6. doi: 10.1016/j.nepr.2018.01.001

Gnani, S., McDonald, H., Islam, S. *et al.* (2014) Patterns of healthcare use among adolescents attending an urban general practitioner-led urgent care centre. *Emergency Medicine Journal*, **31**: 630–6.

Hounsgaard, L., Jensen, A.B., Wilche, J.P. and Dolmer, I. (2013) The nature of nursing practice in rural and remote areas of Greenland. *International Journal of Circumpolar Health*, **72**: 1. doi: 10.3402/ijch.v72i0.20964

Ion, R., Patrick, L., Chouliara, Z. and Barlow, E-L. (2020) Three issues for mental health nurse educators preparing new preregistration programmes. *Mental Health Practice*, **23(3)**: e1453. doi: 10.7748/mhp.2020.e1453

Jack, K. and Hamshire, C. (2019) PLATO: A practice education tool to support learning and professional development. *Nurse Education in Practice*, **37**: 141–5.

McClure, E. and Black, L. (2013) The role of the clinical preceptor: an integrative literature review. *Journal of Nursing Education*, **52(6)**: 335–41.

McKie, A., Baguley, F., Guthrie, C. *et al.* (2012) Exploring clinical wisdom in nursing education. *Nursing Ethics*, **19(2)**: 252–67. doi: 10.1177/0969733011416841

Mental Health Foundation (2013) *Crossing boundaries: Improving integrated care for people with mental health problems.* Final inquiry report, September 2013. Mental Health Foundation. Available at: www.mentalhealth.org.uk/sites/default/files/crossing-boundaries.pdf (accessed 28 September 2020).

NHS England (2014) *Five year forward view.* NHS England. Available at: www.england.nhs.uk/wp-content/uploads/2014/10/5yfv-web.pdf (accessed 13 August 2020).

NHS England (2017) *Next steps on the NHS five year forward view.* NHS England. Available at: www.england.nhs.uk/wp-content/uploads/2017/03/next-steps-on-the-nhs-five-year-forward-view.pdf (accessed 13 August 2020).

Nursing and Midwifery Council (2018) *Future nurse: Standards of proficiency for registered nurses.* NMC. Available at: www.nmc.org.uk/globalassets/sitedocuments/education-standards/future-nurse-proficiencies.pdf (accessed 13 August 2020).

Nursing and Midwifery Council (2020) *Emergency standards for nursing and midwifery education*. NMC. Available at: www.nmc. org.uk/standards-for-education-and-training/emergency-education-standards/ (accessed 13 August 2020).

Office for National Statistics (2011) *Rural/urban classification*. Department for Environment, Food and Rural Affairs. Available at: www.ons.gov.uk/methodology/geography/geographicalproducts/rural urbanclassifications/2011ruralurbanclassification (accessed 13 August 2020).

Olson, A., Reiland, S., Davies, S. and Reitmaier Koehler, A. (2018) Learning about the experience of living with chronic conditions: A framework analysis of nursing students' reflections on their conversations with older adults. *Gerontology and Geriatrics Education*, **39**(3): 295–315. doi: 10.1080/02701960.2016.1247067

Perrin, L., and Scott, S. (2016) Health visitors have much to offer pre-registration child branch student nurses. *Community Practitioner*, **89**(5): 44–7.

Pront, L. and McNeill, L. (2019) Nursing students' perceptions of a clinical learning assessment activity: 'Linking the puzzle pieces of theory to practice'. *Nurse Education in Practice*, **36**: 85–90. doi: 10.1016/j.nepr.2019.03.008

Reynolds, L., Attenborough, J. and Halse, J. (2020) Nurses as educators: creating teachable moments in practice. *Nursing Times*, **116**(2): 25–8.

Roberts, D., Hibberd, P., Lewis, C.A. and Turley, J. (2014) The unique contribution of community clinical nurse specialists in rural Wales. *British Journal of Community Nursing*, **19**(12): 602–7.

van Iersel, M., Latour, C.H.M., de Vos, R., Kirschner, P.A. and Scholte op Reimer, W.J.M. (2016) Nursing students' perceptions of community care and other areas of nursing practice – a review of the literature. *International Journal of Nursing Studies*, **61**: 1–19.

Warwick-Booth, L., Coan, S. and Bagnall, A.M. (2019) Personalised housing support to improve health and well-being: findings from a local pilot programme in Yorkshire, England. *Cities and Health*, **4**(1): 82–93. doi: 10.1080/23748834.2019.1644078

Willis, G.P. (2015) *Shape of caring: A review of the future education and training of registered nurses and care assistants*. Health Education England. Available at: www.hee.nhs.uk/sites/default/files/documents/2348-Shape-of-caring-review-FINAL.pdf (accessed 13 August 2020).

World Health Organization (2018) *Housing and health guidelines.* WHO. Available at: https://apps.who.int/iris/bitstream/handle/ 10665/276001/9789241550376-eng.pdf?ua=1 (accessed 13 August 2020).

Zwakhalen, S.M.G., Hamers, J.P.H., Metzelthin, S.F. *et al.* (2018) Basic nursing care: The most provided, the least evidence based – a discussion paper. *Journal of Clinical Nursing*, 27: 496–2505. doi: 10.1111/jocn.14296

ACTIVITY ANSWER GUIDES

ACTIVITY 1.3

This activity is about creating opportunities for learning that span different educational outcome statements or that combine activities that meet different educational outcomes and perhaps some of the proficiencies in the annexe documents (NMC, 2018). The paper by Reynolds *et al.* (2020) (see *References*) describes how it is possible to create those teachable moments. This might be a good starting point for your thinking.

You may have considered students learning at undergraduate and postgraduate levels; their knowledge base will be different in terms of the level of their thinking but their psychomotor application of the skill carried out as an action might be very different. You might want to think about how you would demonstrate a skill-based activity (such as wound care); your demonstration to the students might be the same, but your explanation and level of questioning for the postgraduate student would need to be more detailed and challenging.

ACTIVITY 1.4

This activity asks you to identify the various learning opportunities that could be available for your area. Here are some examples drawn from a range of educational audits encompassing different placement areas. Notice how the lists include psychomotor skills, communication skills and other areas of learning.

Learning opportunities identified by an outpatient department specialising in gynaecological conditions:

Year 1:

- Communication skills: verbal, written, with staff and patients.
- Practice of infection control procedures including aseptic non-touch technique (ANTT)/hand washing

- Basic clinical observations
- Follow the patient pathway from initial consultation through to procedures in theatre
- Shadowing of nurse specialist to gain an understanding of their role
- Experience specimen collection and procedure
- Chaperone experience
- Be involved with team working
- Gain insight to problems with early pregnancy.

Years 2 and 3:
- Develop communication skills, specifically the breaking of bad news
- Supporting patients in their care, promoting their dignity and respecting their autonomy
- Learning about strategies used to manage situations where a patient's wishes conflict with recommended nursing care or treatment plans
- Correctly undertaking, interpreting and acting on findings from clinical observations
- Follow the patient pathway from initial consultation through to procedures in theatre; be able to discuss with your mentor how and why these pathways are organised and managed
- Learning the relevant investigations and treatment management prior to surgical decisions
- Shadowing of nurse specialist; be able to discuss how they manage their own caseload
- Chaperone experience
- Experience of specimen collection procedures
- Recovery of patients post procedure, under supervision
- Take part in the day-to-day running of the clinics, under supervision
- Co-ordinate clinics, under supervision
- Active involvement in clinics, e.g. colposcopy, under supervision
- Gain insight into problems with early pregnancy
- Opportunities to develop knowledge of and participate in health promotion, e. g. obesity, smoking.

The following learning opportunities have been identified by a team from preoperative assessment clinic, which is nurse led:

Year 1:
- Communication skills: including providing clear instructions
- Infection prevention and control by practising ANTT/hand washing
- Obtaining and accurate recording vital signs

- Self-directed study, e.g. library work
- Spoke placements.

Year 2:
- Communication skills, including providing reassurance and alleviating anxiety
- Infection prevention and control by practising ANTT/hand washing
- Obtaining and accurate recording vital signs, escalating concerns appropriately if outside the normal range
- Providing teaching sessions to peers and colleagues and providing explanations to patients and families
- Spoke placements.

Anonymised educational audit identifying learning opportunities:

XXXXXXXXXXX offers a range of placement opportunities which are relevant to community and acute placement. The services offered are as follows:
1. Step-down care for older adults who are admitted with a variety of medical conditions on XXXXX (male medical) and XXXXX (female) wards
2. Rehabilitation for those who are admitted from the acute sector of XXXXXXX
3. Day treatments services for those with ongoing treatment needs.

The XXXXXXXXXX unit is a nurse-led outpatient healthcare facility which provides a local facility for people requiring treatment/intervention for chronic disease, e.g. intravenous (IV) infusions, venesection and blood transfusion.

The XXXXXXXXXX unit provides a service for people requiring short-term IV therapy on an outpatient basis for acute illness, e.g. IV antibiotics for cellulitis.

The following patients may be referred to the XXXXXXXXX unit and require nursing care:
- Patients who require initiation, titration and monitoring of treatment for chronic disease e.g. ACE inhibitor titration, beta blocker initiation and titration for heart failure
- Patients for phase 3 cardiac rehabilitation
- Patients undergoing intermittent IV therapy for chronic disease, e.g. rheumatology, osteoporosis, ulcerative colitis, Crohn's disease

- Patients requiring short-term IV therapy, e.g. once-daily IV antibiotics for short-term acute illness including via a peripherally inserted central catheter (PICC)
- Patients requiring other procedures such as venesection/iron infusion
- In addition to this, the unit also facilitates multidisciplinary clinics including movement disorder, falls, cardiac rehabilitation and heart failure
- The XXXXXXXXXX unit is led by a senior nurse with advanced clinical assessment skills and an independent prescribing qualification
- The senior nurse is supported by three registered nurses and two healthcare assistants
- The Unit works closely with specialist nurses in Parkinson's disease, osteoporosis, rheumatology and diabetes.

The XXXXXXXXXX unit provides:
- Multidisciplinary falls clinic (XXX morning)
- Phase 3 cardiac rehabilitation
- Nurse-led heart failure clinic, including optimisation of treatment, monitoring, rehabilitation, health education and advice on self-management for patients and carers
- Telehealth monitoring
- Day-case blood transfusion
- IV therapies for people with chronic disease, e.g. osteoporosis, rheumatoid arthritis, ulcerative colitis, chronic kidney disease
- Administration of IV therapy via PICC/Hickman or mid-lines
- IV iron infusion
- IV therapies for uncomplicated short-term illness, e.g. IV antibiotics for cellulitis
- Nurse-led venesection
- Students will have the opportunity to gain knowledge, understanding and proficiency in the following:
  - How the XXXXXXXXXX unit supports the provision of care in the primary care sector
  - How a nurse-led clinic operates and the accountability of those nurses within the clinic and the responsibilities they assume
  - Participation in a range of clinics: falls assessment, cardiac rehabilitation, heart failure, Parkinson's clinic, rheumatology and diabetes
  - Observing the preparation of IV therapies to include drug calculations and mixing/additives

- Observe the process of independent prescribing
- Assess the patient during the process of IV therapy
- Understand the risk of adverse reaction to IV and the emergency response required
- The ongoing assessment of patients as their care needs change with each visit
- Completion of the documentation
- MDT team meetings with XXXXXXXXXX nursing, medical and ancillary staff.

General learning opportunities:
1. Orientation to the delivery of care in the secondary care/community hospital setting
2. Understand and apply the requirements of the NMC and their implications for practice
3. Understand and comply with local policy and guidelines with regards to uniform and comportment, reporting of sickness/non-attendance for duty, and the provision of nursing care
4. Competence in the taking and recording of vital signs to include BP, pulse, temperature and respiratory rate
5. Understand and gain proficiency in the principles of standard precautions, hand washing and other infection control measures to include:
   a. Hand washing technique and the appropriate use of gel agents
   b. Appropriate use of aprons and gloves when providing care
   c. Infection control mechanisms for those with infectious conditions such as *Clostridium difficile*, methicillin-resistant *Staphylococcus aureus* (MRSA), etc.
6. Proficiency in provision of personalised nursing care to include:
   a. Elimination needs of ambulant patients
   b. Cleaning of commodes and other toileting aids
   c. Assisting with personal cleansing and dressing as required while promoting and maintaining independence
7. Competence at manual handling and mobilising patients to include:
   a. The practice of safe manual handling techniques
   b. Assisting registered nurses or AHPs with the assessment of a patient's ability to mobilise and the aids needed/falls assessment
   c. Assisting patients to mobilise as required using appropriate aids
8. Understand and gain proficiency at completing person-centred nursing assessments and relevant nursing care documentation to include:
   a. The use and completion of the nursing process to document care

    b. The use of nursing assessment using relevant tools to assist with the diagnosis of care required

    c. Develop the art of assessing patients using non-objective means such as sight, touch and intuition

9. Understand the process of medication management and become proficient in the administration of medication to include:

    a. Understand the NMC Medication Management Standards and their application to practice

    b. Understand the standards for medication administration to include the six rights of medication administration

    c. Be able to undertake accurate drug dosage calculations and administer correctly under supervision

    d. Understand the role of the nurse as the last point in which an error can be prevented

    e. Understand the contraindications for the administration of prescribed medication

    f. Understand the rights of a competent individual to refuse medication

    g. Understand the pharmacology and pharmokinetics of medication

    h. Understand the role of the pharmacist in maintaining safe medication management

    i. Understand the requirements and processes of adverse incident reporting in the event of a medication error

10. Gain an understanding of the conditions treated within the XXXXXXXXXX unit and the impact this has on the ability of the patient to be independent and self-caring to include:

    a. The aetiology of conditions and the impact on mobility, speech and safe swallow and ability to self-care

    b. Understand the aims and outcomes of the XXXXXXXXXX unit to enable patients to be treated as outpatients

    c. Understand the treatment regimens for each condition, taking into account patient preference and be able to participate in the delivery of same

11. Gain proficiency in communicating effectively with older adults with hearing and sight loss to include:

    a. Understanding the importance of effective communication with patients in the healthcare setting

    b. Understand and use effective non-verbal methods to communicate effectively

    c. Understand the physical and environmental barriers to effective communication and how to attend to these as appropriate to the situation

    d. Understand the role of documentation as a means of communication within the healthcare team

    e. Understand the requirements of confidentiality and how this applies to those assisting with the care of the patient, the MDT, family members

    f. Understand how the Carer's Strategy requires the sharing of some information with carers so that safe and effective care can be provided while adhering to common law, statutory and professional requirements

    g. Understand the requirement of General Data Protection Regulation (GDPR) and the Caldecott requirements with regard to the storing and sharing of data/patient information

12. Understand the requirement to maintain the dignity of all patients at all times to include:

    a. Speaking appropriately to patients at all times and learning how to respond appropriately to those who are upset, disorientated or confused

    b. Ensuring that all patients receiving assistance with personal hygiene or toileting are provided with as much privacy as is possible and also the opportunity to decline assistance if wished

    c. Adhere to local and professional guidelines which are intended to set the standards required to maintain dignity

    d. Understand the processes of reporting care that compromise a patient's dignity

13. Understand the legal and ethical dimensions of nursing to include:

    a. The ethical, legal and professional requirements of gaining consent prior to the delivery of any care or treatment

    b. Understand the rights of a competent patient to refuse treatment

    c. Understand the process of assessing the capacity of a patient

    d. Understand the legal requirements of the Mental Capacity Act and making best interest decisions for those who lack capacity

    e. Understand legal provision with regards to proxy decision-making and the way in which a Lasting Power of Attorney (LPA) is appointed, their role, and also how this person should be involved in best interest decision-making

    f. Understand the legal requirements of ensuring that independent mental capacity advocates are involved in treatment decisions to change or withdraw treatment or to change the residence of patients

     g. Understand the meaning of a 'do not attempt resuscitation' (DNAR) order, when it is appropriate and who should complete this directive

     h. Understand the implication of a DNAR should a patient sustain a cardiorespiratory arrest

14. Understand the causes of a cardiorespiratory arrest and the requirements of basic life support to include:
     a. Understanding the requirement to call for assistance prior to commencing cardiopulmonary resuscitation (CPR)
     b. Understand and assist with CPR as required
     c. If not involved in the CPR activity use communication skills to attend to patients within the immediate vicinity

15. Gain proficiency in, and understanding of, clinical governance strategies and local policy to include:
     a. Use of evidence-based practice in the clinical setting
     b. Identifying best practice for ward speciality
     c. Role of NICE/NSF in care provision/decision-making
     d. Management of risk and the reporting of adverse events
     e. Reporting of near miss or adverse events.

Approaches to education:
- Induction pack and guidance about the student experience
- Numerous opportunities, open to challenge and questions and evaluating care
- Time devoted to the assessment process, including an initial, mid-point and final assessment/interview
- Using NMC standards for learning and assessment, and guidance available at unit level in supervisor/assessor resource file
- Orientation/induction booklets
- Resource file with current articles, evidence, research and papers that students can read on the unit
- DVDs, videos etc. available
- Students involved in ward meetings
- A suggestion book is available for students to give suggestions/feedback for improving the learning environment
- Students are given the opportunity to work with and have supervision from members of the MDT to identify and better understand their role, responsibilities and specialised area of practice
- Practice supervisors promote reflections on experience
- Practical teaching on one-to-one, formal and informal sessions

- Information is shared and learning opportunities are created and used well
- Provide learning opportunities through case conferences, case notes, nursing notes, learning by doing, observing other staff, talking with patients and carers.

Other learning opportunities:
- Informal: colleagues, learning pack, books, articles, information displayed on ward, British Heart Foundation booklets
- Formal: regular teaching on the ward by medical reps and ward nursing staff
- Additionally, staff can arrange for you to spend time in the other areas of cardiology (CCU, cardiac centre and cath lab, cardiac rehabilitation) and also with other members of the MDT as appropriate.

ACTIVITY 1.6

"Standard 2.10: provide information in accessible ways to help people understand and make decisions about their health, life choices, illness and care". You might consider making information available through easy-read guides, or through pictures. For a good example, see the easy-read guides provided by Mencap:
www.mencap.org.uk/advice-and-support/coronavirus-covid-19/coronavirus-guidance-help-you-stay-safe-and-well

and visual posters:
https://assets.publishing.service.gov.uk/government/uploads/system/uploads/attachment_data/file/869144/Self-isolation_poster_for_patients.pdf

ACTIVITY 1.7

Examples of other hard-to-reach groups might include the oldest old (over 85 years), people from black and ethnic minority groups, people identifying as lesbian, bisexual, gay or transsexual, for example. Geography may play a part in terms of being hard to reach; or there may be social, economic or political reasons why groups or populations might be hard to reach. Social exclusion = the oldest old, economic exclusion = rough sleepers or the homeless who cannot afford to travel to reach health services, and political exclusion = refugees and asylum seekers, for example.

There might be specific services set up designed to reach out to these groups; if these exist in your areas, as a supervisor it is important for you to be aware of these services, so that you can arrange for students to spend time there, learning about these hard-to-reach groups.

ACTIVITY 1.8

You might consider discussing with the student opportunities for promoting health and preventing ill health; whether the individual is an inappropriate attender, and should be directed to alternative services, or if the adolescent woman is a sex worker, whether that changes the nature of the consultation? You could direct the student to find evidence related to the role of the nurse in health education and promotion in emergency settings.

CHAPTER 2

DEVELOPING THE EDUCATION TEAM

Jacqueline Leigh and Debbie Roberts

2.1 INTRODUCTION

This chapter explores the culture for practice learning through developing the education team. The education team will of course include the three new roles outlined by the Nursing and Midwifery Council (NMC): **practice supervisor, practice assessor** and **academic assessor;** but it has long been recognised that students learn from everyone that they meet in the clinical learning environment. This chapter therefore discusses the importance of building a culture where learning and practice development is everyone's business.

After reading this chapter you will be able to:

- Identify and discuss the factors that make an effective practice learning environment
- Understand the impact that the learning culture has on promoting effective student supervision and assessment
- Explore the NMC *Part 2: Standards for supervision and assessment* and discuss the role of the education team in delivering quality supervision and assessment where you work
- Understand the role of practice supervisor, practice assessor and academic assessor in supporting the student to meet NMC programme requirements.

The Nursing and Midwifery Council (NMC) in its new standards framework for nurse education (NMC, 2018b) makes clear that an effective practice learning environment is one which provides opportunities for meaningful learning experiences that contribute to a student meeting their programme learning outcomes and NMC proficiencies. An effective practice learning environment therefore requires a learning culture that prioritises the safety of people, including patients, carers, students and educators, and enables the values of *The Code* (NMC, 2018e) to be upheld. The culture within an effective practice learning environment should value learning, and all people within the learning environment should understand their role in enabling learning. Creating an effective learning environment that includes providing students with quality supervision and assessment involves ensuring that the personnel are equipped with the right knowledge and skills to support students to achieve programme learning outcomes and NMC proficiencies. The effective learning environment is not something that is developed just for students; learning should be embedded throughout the area and should be everyone's business.

This chapter will first explore the global standards for initial education of professional nurses and midwives. The factors that make an effective practice learning environment will be identified and discussed. This will include understanding the impact that the learning culture has on promoting effective student supervision and assessment. Through engaging in a series of activities, you will explore the NMC *Part 2: Standards for supervision and assessment* to raise awareness of the crucial role of the education team in delivering quality supervision and assessment. This exploration will increase your knowledge of the NMC roles of practice supervisor, practice assessor and academic assessor as well as other roles involved in student learning from within the practice learning environment.

2.2 GLOBAL STANDARDS FOR THE INITIAL EDUCATION OF PROFESSIONAL NURSES AND MIDWIVES

The diversity of initial preparation of nurses and midwives is highlighted in the World Health Organization (WHO) *Global standards for the initial education of professional nurses and midwives* (WHO, 2009) which calls for the standard to be agreed globally at degree level. The WHO does acknowledge, however, that many countries will be working towards this standard. The global standards aim to provide an opportunity for investment in those areas that raise the standard of initial education of nurses and midwives, with the person-centred curriculum being firmly rooted in academic education institutions or universities. The WHO *State of the world's nursing 2020: investing in education, jobs and leadership* (WHO, 2020) calls for the investment in the massive acceleration of nursing education. This includes faculty, infrastructure and students – to address global needs, meet domestic demand, and respond to changing technologies and advancing models of integrated health and social care.

In the UK there is the relatively new role of the **nursing associate** which also requires the student (**trainee nursing associate**) to undertake a programme validated by a university. For the purpose of this chapter the term 'student' will encompass student nurse, midwife and trainee nursing associate.

It is important to remember that universities, whether providing undergraduate nursing or midwifery programmes, cannot achieve this education standard alone; students also need to learn from the experience of being in a clinical or practice learning environment. Close working relationships are therefore required with clinical practice and qualified nurses, midwives and nursing associates who support, supervise and assess students to achieve clinical learning standards and NMC programme-specific proficiencies (NMC, 2018a, b, c, d). The principles enshrined within the global standards are quite clear in that the interaction between the student and the client should be the "primary focus of quality education and care" (p. 19), further emphasising the importance of clinically based supervision and assessment. Clinical learning is woven throughout many of the global standards. Students should be provided with "supervised clinical learning experiences" (standard 3.2.4) in order to develop "clinical reasoning, problem solving and critical thinking" (standard 3.1.7).

The new NMC (2018b, c, d) standards also support the notion of learning being embedded within the real world of clinical practice. Indeed, within UK programmes leading to registration as a nurse, midwife or nursing associate, students spend time learning in the clinical practice environment and university classroom in equal measure. Students are expected to work alongside NMC registrants and other professionals who share their craft knowledge and help the student to learn. It is recognised that all healthcare professionals and indeed patients have a wealth of knowledge that should be passed on to students. The relationship between the supervisor and the student is crucially important, having a direct impact on the student experience.

This next part of the chapter will explore what is meant by the practice learning environment.

☑ ACTIVITY 2.1

Reflect on a time when you engaged in a learning activity that took place from within the practice learning environment. From your experience identify three factors that impacted on your learning.

This is a personal reflective activity, so no answer guide is provided.

2.3 THE QUALITY PRACTICE LEARNING ENVIRONMENT

2.3.1 *Exploring factors that create an effective practice learning environment*

Practice-based learning is a term associated with undertaking learning while on placement. Indeed, to be considered safe and effective, the NMC (2018b) states that a learning environment must have the right people in place to supervise and support students. Who the right people are will differ depending on the practice learning circumstance of the student, and may include the combination of university and practice staff. This means that practice learning teams can look different depending on the type of learning with which the student will engage.

There is a wealth of literature that explores those factors that make an effective learning environment and if not in place can negatively impact learning and following completion of *Activity 2.1* you will have identified some of these.

For example, as far back as the inception of the Florence Nightingale School of Nursing in 1890, the matron and ward sister together with the doctor played a prominent role in creating the conducive clinical learning environment whereby probationers (students) relied on 'on the job' training to learn the craft of nursing. The key to promoting the conducive clinical learning environment here is having somebody who shows an interest in student learning and development, and role models the behaviours expected of a competent, caring and compassionate nurse. The philosophy of the 'interested person' remains true today and to create the effective clinical learning environment requires great leadership skills by all involved in practice learning and this is explored in more detail in *Chapter 9*. For example, the RCN (2017) has developed a toolkit for helping students get the best from their practice placements, providing the evidence of what makes an effective practice learning environment. The toolkit is specifically designed for use with the previous educational standards, but nonetheless there are transferable ideas. Evidence includes strong leadership from the senior leadership team who value education through, for example, providing time and resources for those with a responsibility for student learning to attend events or complete online learning activities.

You can download the RCN (2017) toolkit *Helping students get the best from their practice placements* via their website here: www.rcn.org.uk/professional-development/publications/pub-006035

Another factor that helps to create the effective clinical learning environment is recognising that to learn the craft of nursing or midwifery might mean engaging in learning in non-traditional environments. Diverse learning environments may include engaging with voluntary and third sector organisations. This is particularly relevant when thinking about person-centred care and social prescribing opportunities for people. Equally, valuing service users and carers as experts, and the contribution that they can make when providing feedback on the student's practice and development, promotes the quality clinical learning environment.

Engaging in a practice learning environment that values education is quite often referred to as an environment that has the right learning culture. This is explored in more detail next.

2.3.2 What is the learning culture?

The culture of the clinical learning environment and the quality of clinical supervision are inextricably linked. In an interesting study conducted across Finland, Pitkänen *et al.* (2018, p. 143) emphasised the importance of "individualized and goal-oriented supervision in which the student had a named supervisor and where supervision was completed as planned in a positive environment that supported learning had a significant impact on students' learning". The study showed the significant effect of positive supervision and positive supervisory relationships on student learning. They go so far as to say that "clinical learning consists of two parts: the learning environment and supervision" (Pitkänen *et al.*, 2018, p. 144).

There is no doubt that the clinical milieu is full of rich learning experiences and that learning is more meaningful if the learner actively participates; this is why it is so important for each clinical learning area to identify the range of opportunities for learning. The learning culture then is the way in which nurses and other members of the multidisciplinary team (MDT) within that environment concern themselves with supporting learning in others and their own personal engagement with learning. Learning within clinical practice is not limited to students observing or engaging with qualified staff. It has long been known that others in the clinical area (and beyond) play a valid part in supporting student learning (Andrews and Roberts, 2003). The culture of clinical learning means that everyone makes learning their business; there is a conscious effort to engage with learning through practice development initiatives to personal learning and the supporting or teaching of others.

The primary role of the student in clinical practice is to learn. However, the primary role of the nurse in clinical practice is to care for patients, and these two elements sometimes clash as nurses experience emotional conflict between the two. An effective clinical learning culture considers this dissonance and provides assistance for nurses to teach and support the learning of students and others. Henderson and Eaton (2013) call for senior leadership personnel to establish a culture where the value of teaching and learning in practice is recognised and fostered by the entire team. For example, rosters should be considered so that learner and student and what they term as the 'learning guide' can work together. Every opportunity is perceived and used as a potential learning opportunity; learning guides step back from actually carrying out a task in order to facilitate the learner to undertake the task with support and feedback. However, Henderson and Eaton (2013) acknowledge that this takes time, which should be taken into account, and the workload of the learning guide should be altered accordingly. The WHO (2020) advocates the need to strengthen both current and future nurse leadership, ensuring that nurses have an influential role in health policy formulation and decision-making, and contribute to the effectiveness of health and social care systems. This leadership should also be used to influence practice learning for all students.

ACTIVITY 2.2

In terms of developing a supporting learning culture within a clinical placement it might be useful to undertake the following reflective exercise suggested by Cranton (2016, p. 145):

    What is my purpose in being an educator?
    How do I see the learners I work with?
    What constraints or resistances influence my practice?

This is a personal reflective activity, so no answer guide is provided.

Following this activity, you might want to compare your thoughts with the Royal College of Nursing Wales Education Strategy (2016): *The future of nursing education in Wales*. You can access the report through their website here:

www.rcn.org.uk/about-us/our-influencing-work/policy-briefings/education-strategy

The report highlights the important role of education (learning in clinical practice) as a driver for enhancing patient experiences. The report also makes recommendations for skill mix.

2.4 NMC *FUTURE NURSE: STANDARDS OF PROFICIENCY FOR REGISTERED NURSES*; AND *REALISING PROFESSIONALISM: PART 3: STANDARDS FOR EDUCATION AND TRAINING*

Following a 2-year process that included consulting and working alongside key stakeholder groups such as students, educators, health professionals, charities and patient groups from across the UK, the NMC launched its *Future nurse: Standards of proficiency for registered nurses* (NMC, 2018a) and *Realising professionalism: Standards for education and training* (NMC, 2018b, c, d). These compulsory standards must be used in nurse education curricula by approved education institutions (universities). The standards for education and training consist of three parts that are summarised in *Box 2.1*.

Box 2.1: Summary of the NMC standards for education and training

> **Part 1: Standards framework for nursing and midwifery education** This document is split into five sections that underpin nurse education and training:
> 1. Learning culture
> 2. Educational governance and quality
> 3. Student learning and empowerment
> 4. Educators and assessors
> 5. Curricula and assessment.
>
> **Part 2: Standards for student supervision and assessment** These set out the expectations for the learning, support, supervision and assessment (of theory and practice) of students in the practice environment.
>
> **Part 3: Standards for pre-registration nursing programmes** These set out the legal requirements for all pre-registration nursing education programmes.

Collectively, these documents, together with *Future nurse: Standards of proficiency for registered nurses* (NMC, 2018a), specify the knowledge and skills registered nurses must demonstrate when caring for people of all ages and across all care settings; these reflect what the public can expect nurses and midwives to know and be able to do to ensure the delivery of safe, compassionate and effective care. A key message, and something that maintains continuity with the preceding pre-registration standards (NMC, 2010), is the fundamental requirement for partnerships between universities and healthcare organisations to provide the practice-based learning for nursing students:

> *"Universities are responsible for working with practice learning partners to manage the quality of their educational programmes. Overall responsibility for the day-to-day management of the quality of any educational programme lies*

with a university in partnership with practice learning partners who provide opportunities for practice experience to nursing and midwifery students". (NMC, 2018b, p. 4)

This above statement clearly emphasises the need for developing the education team that includes membership of people from both the university and the practice partner organisations.

The remaining part of the chapter will focus on the *Part 2: Standards for student supervision and assessment* (NMC, 2018c), exploring content implications for practice learning, supervision and assessment.

2.5 NMC *PART 2: STANDARDS FOR STUDENT SUPERVISION AND ASSESSMENT* – IMPLICATIONS FOR PRACTICE TEACHING, LEARNING AND ASSESSMENT

The NMC (2018c) is proud of its new standards, which provide greater opportunities for nurses and midwives, as well as other registered health and care professionals, to support and improve the quality of student learning. Part 2 describes changes to the way that students are supported in clinical practice with the NMC, shifting focus not only from the pivotal role of mentor but introducing three new roles: that of **practice supervisor, practice assessor** and **academic assessor.**

When thinking about the three roles, the NMC makes clear that, under normal circumstances, individuals cannot be practice supervisor and practice assessor for the same student. In addition, practice assessors are not simultaneously the practice supervisor and academic assessor for the same student. These NMC requirements should be considered when reading this chapter.

The assessment is to be conducted by a registered nurse, midwife or nursing associate with suitable equivalent qualifications for the programme the student is undertaking, and who is not on a temporary register. The roles of supervisor and assessor are separate, and individuals cannot be both supervisor and assessor for the same student, although they can perform both roles for different students.

Each of the three roles is discussed in turn, with this chapter applying the NMC (2018a, b, c, d) standards.

2.5.1 *Practice supervisor*

Practice supervision enables students to learn and safely achieve proficiency and autonomy in their professional role. In Part 2 of the standards, the

NMC describes the roles and responsibilities of the **practice supervisor** and these are summarised in *Box 2.2.* Practice supervisors will supervise students learning in practice who are working towards achievement of the programme learning outcomes and proficiencies.

Box 2.2: The practice supervisor's role and responsibilities

- Serve as role models for safe and effective practice in line with **The Code** (NMC, 2018e)
- Support learning in line with their scope of practice to enable the student to meet their proficiencies and programme outcomes
- Support and supervise students, providing feedback on their progress towards, and achievement of, proficiencies and skills
- Have current knowledge and experience of the area in which they are providing support, supervision and feedback
- Receive ongoing support to participate in the practice learning of students

The NMC makes very clear that all NMC registered nurses and midwives are capable of supervising students, providing they have been prepared and supported to take up their role and have up-to-date knowledge and experience relevant to the student they are supervising. Serving as role models for safe and effective practice, the NMC is clearly placing responsibility for supervising student learning with every registrant in any practice-learning environment.

The NMC is not explicit about the number of practice supervisors allocated to the student per clinical placement, therefore providing education teams with the flexibility to promote practice supervisor models whereby the student can learn from more than one NMC registrant working in the practice supervisor role at any one time.

Practice supervision enables students to learn about all aspects of the nursing and midwifery role. Through students learning in safe environments (under supervision) and over the duration of the pre-registration programme, this ensures that they become autonomous practitioners who are able to exercise their full professional role. In other words, the practice supervisor guides the student towards being an independent learner.

For the first time the NMC in the *Part 2: Standards for student supervision and assessment* is acknowledging that other professionals also have a role to play in the supervision of student learning in clinical practice. The NMC makes clear that health and social care registrants of all the professional bodies should contribute to the learning and development of nursing students (NMC, 2018c, p. 6). However, practice supervisors must be registered with a professional regulator, for example the General Medical Council or the Health and Care Professions Council. While health and social care professionals who are not registered with a professional regulator cannot be practice supervisors, they may still contribute to nursing and midwifery education. Such roles include phlebotomists or teachers (in a primary or secondary school).

So, it is vitally important that as an NMC registrant you think about what your role might be within your clinical area. You might be one of a team of supervisors that contributes to student learning; so, you should also consider ways in which you will meet with those individuals and discuss student progression. Of course, many registered nurses and midwives will have taken on the role of mentor for students. Mentorship is a system of teaching and assessing student nurses and midwives in the UK, under the preceding NMC standards for education (NMC, 2010). The roles of mentor and practice supervisor do share some similarities but all students exiting NMC-accredited programmes that have been validated against the new NMC standards will be suitably prepared for their supervisory role during their pre-registration programme. The preparation may look different in different programmes and across different universities and healthcare organisations.

Here is one example of a practice supervisor and assessor guide developed by Health Education and Improvement Wales (2018):

https://heiw.nhs.wales/files/once-for-wales-docs/all-wales-practice-supervisor-assessor-guide/

Preparation should meet NMC requirements and should be developed collaboratively between the university and its practice learning partners to ensure that practice supervisors receive ongoing support to prepare, reflect and develop for effective supervision and contribution to student learning and assessment; and have understanding of the proficiencies and programme outcomes they are supporting students to achieve. Particularly as students prepare for NMC registration, it is important that the practice supervisory role responsibilities are explored, with students developing strategies to reflect and identify their own learning needs around the role requirements. The practice supervisory role is also a key component of healthcare organisation preceptorship programmes for NMC newly registered practitioners.

Those registrants that have previously taken on the role of mentor or sign-off mentor may require some additional training or updating in order to enable them to take on the new supervisory role. These arrangements will be determined locally, so you might need to check what the local arrangements are within your area of work. What you may notice is how the preparation for the practice supervisor role may be less prescriptive than previously experienced when preparing for the role of mentor or sign-off mentor.

To help you to prepare for the role, or evidence that you meet role requirements, the requirements have been categorised into knowledge, skills and behaviours and these are presented in *Table 2.1*. It would be useful to reflect on those knowledge, skills and behaviours that you can currently evidence and for you to consider any identified gaps or ongoing learning as a continuing professional development need, exploring with your line manager and healthcare organisation the development opportunities that are available to you.

Table 2.1: Knowledge, skills, behaviours and role preparation required by the practice supervisor

Knowledge	Skills	Behaviours
Have current knowledge and experience of the area in which they are providing support, supervision and feedback	Support learning in line with their scope of practice to enable the student to meet their proficiencies and programme outcomes	Serve as role models for safe and effective practice in line with their code of conduct
Understand the proficiencies and programme outcomes they are supporting students to achieve	Support and supervise students, providing feedback on their progress towards, and achievement of, proficiencies and skills	Role model behaviours demonstrating that they are receiving ongoing support to participate in the practice learning of students
	Contribute to the student's record of achievement by periodically recording relevant observations on the conduct, proficiency and achievement of the students they are supervising	Apply leadership skills to receive ongoing support to prepare, reflect and develop for effective supervision of, and contribution to, student learning and assessment
	Contribute to student assessments to inform decisions for progression	
	Create sufficient opportunities to engage with practice assessors and academic assessors to share relevant observations on the conduct, proficiency and achievement of the students they are supervising	
	Appropriately raise and respond to student conduct and competence concerns and be supported in doing so	

Table 2.2 provides an example of development opportunities that can help you to prepare and maintain your knowledge, skills and behaviours.

Universities will adopt different ways to demonstrate that practice supervisors are suitably prepared. One way is to use the self-declaration form whereby practice supervisors self-declare that they meet NMC knowledge, skills and behaviours role requirements. This information is collated through university and practice partner healthcare organisations' electronic systems, with the information used as part of university NMC quality assurance processes. It will be useful for you to find out how you will demonstrate to your organisation that you have met and are maintaining proficiency in the role.

Table 2.2: Example of development opportunities to help prepare and maintain practice supervisor knowledge, skills and behaviours

Knowledge	Skills	Behaviours
Read and become familiar with the NMC standards for student supervision and assessment	Workshop attendance (face-to-face or online)	Use reflection to examine your own practice and ongoing development, using revalidation and personal development review to support the process
Find out about proficiencies and programme outcomes you are supporting students to achieve from the university and NMC website	Simulation-based education	Identify who will support and guide you in your role and how this support will be accessed
	Undertake a preparation programme developed collaboratively between the university and practice partner healthcare organisations	
	Undertake professional development activities, utilising relevant educational resources	

✎ ACTIVITY 2.3

If you have not already done so, download the NMC (2018c) *Standards for student supervision and assessment*:
www.nmc.org.uk/standards-for-education-and-training/standards-for-student-supervision-and-assessment/

Compile a list of all the professional groups that contribute to patient care where you work.
     This is a personal reflective activity, so no answer guide is provided.

From your list start to think about how students might be able to work and learn alongside those professional groups in a meaningful way: for example, are there particular skills that these individuals use that are also included within the NMC standards and proficiencies? Use *Table 2.3* to help with completion of this activity.

What, if any, preparation or mechanisms need to be put in place to support the development of the learning environment where learning becomes everyone's business?

Offered below is *Scenario 2.1* about Jan, a senior physiotherapist. Read the case study and then complete *Activity 2.4* that explores how Jan can support student learning when working as the practice supervisor.

🗁 SCENARIO 2.1

Jan is a senior physiotherapist working on an intensive care unit (ICU). Physiotherapists, as part of a wider multidisciplinary team, play an important role in the patient's recovery within intensive care settings.

> *"Patients in an ICU may require mechanical ventilation to help their breathing; however, this can lead to pulmonary complications. Respiratory physiotherapy involves early mobilisation where possible, repositioning patients within bed to optimise respiratory function, and utilising manual techniques or the manipulation of ventilator settings to clear lung secretions that build up within the lungs, when mobility and consequently deep breathing is limited. This helps to reduce the risk of pulmonary issues."* (Wainwright *et al.*, 2017).

Physiotherapists will use a range of knowledge, skills and techniques to assess respiratory function. In particular they listen to the chest during a process known as auscultation to assess airflow through the trachea and bronchial tree; they are listening for normal and abnormal breath sounds that might suggest infection (pneumonia) or disease. Jan attends a ventilated patient in the ICU called Robert, who is recovering from recent major cardiac surgery. Jan needs to assess whether Robert is developing pneumonia, which can be associated with ventilated patients. Jan uses her knowledge of anatomy and physiology of the respiratory system; she looks for key landmarks to know where to place the stethoscope in order to hear breath sounds and use her clinical knowledge to assess if what she hears is normal or abnormal. The information gained through the respiratory assessment is combined with Robert's wider observations: his clinical vital signs (blood pressure, body temperature, oxygen saturation and pulse rate) and general condition for Jan to build up a clinical picture.

☑ ACTIVITY 2.4

Think about how and why you would enable a second-year student to work with Jan, and what knowledge Jan can help the student to learn or apply to Robert, together with the standards and proficiencies Jan might be able to help the student to observe, rehearse and practise? As a practice supervisor, how will you work with Jan to ensure that she understands where the student is in their learning journey, the knowledge and skills that the student may already have but need to apply to practice or build on further and how the three of you might agree the learning outcomes required, and how these might be assessed?

Now consider if the student or indeed the patient is a children's nursing student/child or learning disability nursing student/has a learning difficulty? How might this impact on the learning and teaching?

An answer guide is included at the end of the chapter.

2.5.1.1 *Student supervision: knowing the student*

Every student is an individual; it is important that as a practice supervisor you understand what programme of learning the student you are supporting is studying. While all pre-registration nurse education programmes in the UK are at a minimum of degree level, some programmes leading to initial qualification may also be at postgraduate or master's level.

☑ ACTIVITY 2.5

Start to think about what students at different academic levels will need when they are on your ward or unit for their clinical placement. You need to be prepared to develop students at all levels, with various previous knowledge, skills set and confidence levels. It may also be useful to refer to *Chapter 3 Activity 3.12* that introduces you to Hersey and Blanchard's Situational Leadership Model, a model that assists you in knowing what level of support or delegation is suitable for each learner. Find out what programmes your partner higher education institution offers and familiarise yourself with the programme documents.

This is a personal reflective activity, so no answer guide is provided.

At different stages of the programme the student will be expected to learn different things. These clinical competencies/proficiencies will be set out in the practice assessment document. The practice assessment document is a collection of relevant documents that will enable students to demonstrate their achievement of the NMC educational standards. The practice assessment document may be part of a portfolio of development that the student is expected to construct over the education programme. The exact nature of the practice assessment document will vary depending on where the students are undertaking their pre-registration nurse education programme. Scotland and Wales both have a national practice assessment document, and some parts of England have also joined together to use the same practice assessment documentation; for example, Pan Greater Manchester adapted from the Pan London document. It is the student's responsibility to keep their practice assessment document and portfolio up to date.

Learning outcomes may relate to knowledge or skills that the student is expected to be able to demonstrate and which you, as the practice supervisor, may be expected to facilitate. This is an important point because the decision about the level of supervision required rests with the **practice supervisor.**

Practice supervisors are expected to provide students with opportunities to observe, rehearse and practise; and it is the responsibility of the practice supervisor to provide feedback to the student regarding progress. This formative feedback can also be called formative assessment. Helminen *et al.* (2016, p. 309) describe formative assessment as: "an ongoing process [which] lasts throughout clinical education based on mentors giving feedback; its purpose is to advise the student toward a goal". Assessment practices are covered in more detail in *Chapter 7*.

You might want to download the paper by Helminen *et al.* (2016) from the reference list, and start to plan the process of providing opportunities for students to observe, rehearse and practice in your area, and how and when you will provide meaningful and regular feedback to the student on their progress. Discussions regarding student progress can be challenging but should always be framed (discussed and clearly documented) in a fair and positive manner; this is discussed further in *Chapter 5* (providing honest feedback and feedforward to facilitate learning) and *Chapter 6*. The practice assessor will utilise the formative assessment as evidence that the student is meeting programme proficiencies and intended learning outcomes. Arrangements should be in place locally for the practice supervisors and assessors to communicate directly with each other to discuss the student's progress.

Because of the success of widening participation strategies across higher education, more students with learning differences and/or disabilities are attending university and accessing nurse education. Neurodiversity is a term used to describe a group of "non-related, cognitive disabilities such as dyslexia, dyscalculia, dyspraxia/DCD, autistic spectrum disorder, Asperger syndrome, Tourette syndrome and attention deficit hyperactivity disorder (ADHD)" (Dalton, 2013, p. 72). It will be important for all those engaging in supporting student learning in clinical practice to think about how to best support students with learning differences and/or other disabilities.

ACTIVITY 2.6

Download the following paper by Tee and Cowen (2012) and start to discuss with your colleagues how you might provide additional skills rehearsal, negotiate shift patterns and support disclosure:

Tee, S. and Cowen, M. (2012) Supporting students with disabilities – Promoting understanding amongst mentors in practice. *Nurse Education in Practice*, **12(1):** 6–10.

This is a group activity, so no answer guide is provided, but *Chapter 8* in this book provides a range of approaches using simulation that might help you to plan for and support students with learning differences.

ACTIVITY 2.7

Earlier in the chapter we introduced the global standards for the initial education of professional nurses. Now that you have explored the role of practice supervisor, we ask you to download *Global standards for the initial education of professional nurses and midwives* (WHO, 2009): www.who.int/hrh/nursing_midwifery/hrh_global_standards_education.pdf

Look at pages 20–29 which contain the various outcomes related to programme graduates; look at section 4.2: Clinical faculty. There are three aspects to the role of clinical faculty; think about your role as a practice supervisor and how you might be meeting these standards, particularly regarding qualifications and your clinical expertise, expectations around supervision and assessment and partnership working.

This is a personal reflective activity, so no answer guide is provided.

2.5.2 *Practice assessor*

Practice assessment is discussed more fully in *Chapter 7* of this book; a brief overview is provided here. Those registrants who have previously taken on the role of mentor or sign-off mentor may require some additional training or updating in order to enable them to take on the role of **practice**

assessor. As with the role of practice supervisor these arrangements will be determined locally, so you might need to check the local arrangements within your area of work. What you may notice is how the preparation for the practice assessor role is less prescriptive than previously experienced when preparing for the role of mentor or sign-off mentor.

In *Part 2: Standards for student supervision and assessment*, the NMC (2018c) describe the roles and responsibilities of the practice assessor and these are summarised in *Box 2.3*.

Box 2.3: Roles and responsibilities of the practice assessor

- Conduct assessments to confirm the student's achievement of proficiencies and programme outcomes for practice learning
- Make assessment decisions that are informed by feedback sought and received from practice supervisors
- Make and record objective, evidence-based assessments on conduct, proficiency and achievement, drawing on student records, direct observations, student self-reflection and other resources
- Work in partnership with the nominated academic assessor to evaluate and recommend the student for progression for each part of the programme, in line with programme standards and local and national policies
- Provide sufficient opportunities for the practice assessor to observe the student periodically across environments in order to inform decisions for assessment and progression

What you will see is how the practice assessor role separates the responsibility for assessing student learning from that of the practice supervisor. By separating out the assessment element of the role, it is hoped that assessment of student knowledge and skill will become more robust and objective. There are elements of the practice assessor role that are similar to the previous role of sign-off mentor and these include the need for robust objective and evidence-based assessment decision-making. The major difference is that the practice assessor is not required to confirm students as having reached the required standard of proficiency for safe and effective practice for entry onto the NMC Register. As you continue through this chapter you will see how this confirmation requirement becomes the role of the academic assessor.

There is an uneasy relationship in terms of what is being assessed between competence, capability, intuition and/or expertise (Roberts, 2011). Assessment should not be a 'snapshot' of the student's development; rather it should confirm "student achievement of proficiencies and programme outcomes for practice learning" (NMC, 2018c, p. 9) across all clinical settings and across potentially a range of practice placements. Therefore, the practice assessor will draw on a range of evidence in partnership with the student, the practice supervisor(s), and others who have participated in the student's learning journey over a period of time, gathering feedback and document evidence in relation to the student's progress. Regular, ongoing communication between the practice supervisor and the practice assessor is paramount to avoid the single, snapshot assessment and different currencies of value being ascribed to nursing practice. Accurate documentation is therefore key. This communication and documentation should be recorded in the practice assessment document.

Practice assessors will require a repertoire of questioning skills in order to gather evidence from a range of individuals, sources and documents associated with student learning. In *Chapter 3* you will explore effective questioning skills. For example, practice assessors using the Socratic questioning method can enhance the assessment process through asking the questions that demonstrate the student's skills around critical thinking and self-reflection.

 TOP TIP

Breaking the role responsibilities into knowledge, skills and behaviours (see *Table 2.3* for an example) can help you to reflect and evidence those that you currently have and consider any gaps and ongoing learning as a continuing professional development need, exploring with your line manager and healthcare organisation the development opportunities that are available to you. *Table 2.3* provides an example of development opportunities that can help you to prepare and maintain your knowledge, skills and behaviours.

Table 2.3: Knowledge, skills, behaviours and role preparation required by the practice assessor

Knowledge	Skills	Behaviours
Maintain current knowledge and expertise relevant for the proficiencies and programme outcomes they are assessing	Conduct assessments to confirm student achievement of proficiencies and programme outcomes for practice learning; conduct objective, evidence-based assessments of students	Role model behaviours demonstrating that they are receiving ongoing support and training to reflect and develop in their role
Understand the student's learning and achievement in theory	Make assessment decisions that are informed by feedback sought and received from practice supervisors	Apply leadership skills to proactively develop their professional practice and knowledge in order to fulfil their role

Table 2.3: (cont'd)

Knowledge	Skills	Behaviours
Knowledge of the assessment process and their role within it	Make and record objective, evidence-based assessments on conduct, proficiency and achievement, drawing on student records, direct observations, student self-reflection and other resources	
	Partnership working with the nominated academic assessor to evaluate and recommend the student for progression for each part of the programme, in line with programme standards and local and national policies	
	Create sufficient opportunities to periodically observe the student across environments in order to inform decisions for assessment and progression	
	Create sufficient opportunities to gather and coordinate feedback from practice supervisors, any other practice assessors and relevant people, in order to be assured about their decisions for assessment and progression	
	Time management and communication skills to communicate, collaborate and manage student progression with academic assessors at scheduled and relevant points in programme structure	
	For students on NMC-approved prescribing programmes support learning in line with the NMC standards for prescribing programmes	
	Demonstrate interpersonal communication skills, relevant to student learning and assessment	
	Provide constructive feedback to facilitate professional development in others (preparation)	

☑ **ACTIVITY 2.8**

Find out what your organisation requires from you in order to demonstrate that you have met and are maintaining proficiency in the role.
This is a personal reflective activity, so no answer guide is provided.

Table 2.4 provides examples of practice assessor development opportunities that can help you to prepare and maintain your knowledge, skills and behaviours.

Table 2.4: *Example of practice assessor development opportunities*

Knowledge	Skills	Behaviours
Read and become familiar with the NMC standards for student supervision and assessment	Workshop attendance (face-to-face or online)	Use reflection to examine your own practice and ongoing development, using revalidation and personal development review to support the process
Find out about proficiencies and programme outcomes you are supporting students to achieve, from the university and NMC website	Simulation-based education	Consider use of testimonies from others to understand your communication skills and partnership working
	Undertake a preparation programme developed collaboratively between the university and practice partner healthcare organisations focusing on the role core skills such as assessment and feedback	Identify who will support and guide you in your role and how this support will be accessed, focusing on areas such as resilience and how you respond to difficult situations around challenging assessment, underperforming students and raising concerns
	Undertake professional development activities, utilising relevant educational resources such as effective application of policies and procedures when making objective assessments or raising concerns about student progress	

2.5.3 Academic assessor

In its new standards, the NMC also introduces the role of the **academic assessor,** a role undertaken by an academic situated in the university. The roles and responsibilities of the academic assessor are identified in *Box 2.4.*

The purpose of the academic assessor role is to collate and confirm student achievement of proficiencies and programme outcomes and recommend the student for progression for each part of the programme, in line with programme standards and local and national policies. The academic assessor takes over from the previous role of the sign-off mentor whose role responsibilities confirmed students as having reached the required standard of proficiency for safe and effective practice for entry onto the NMC Register.

Box 2.4: Roles and responsibilities of the academic assessor

> * Collate and confirm student achievement of proficiencies and programme outcomes in the academic environment for each part of the programme
> * Make and record objective, evidence-based decisions on conduct, proficiency and achievement, and recommendations for progression, drawing on student records and other resources
> * Work in partnership with a nominated practice assessor to evaluate and recommend the student for progression for each part of the programme, in line with programme standards and local and national policies
> * Have an understanding of the student's learning and achievement in practice
> * Communicate and collaborate with the practice assessor at relevant points in the student's programme
> * Academic assessors are not simultaneously the practice supervisor and practice assessor for the same student

The NMC is clear that the student must be assigned to a different nominated academic assessor as they progress through each part of the programme, and that the academic assessor will understand and confirm the proficiencies and programme outcomes that the student they confirm is aiming to achieve. Each university programme will assign a different meaning to a 'part' of the programme and it is recommended that you find out this meaning for the programmes that you will confirm. For example, the 'part' in a 3-year undergraduate nursing programme may be the end of each year.

The NMC does not prescribe an academic assessor model. Described below is the model applied to pre-registration nursing, midwifery and trainee nursing associate programmes at the University of Salford.

University of Salford academic assessor model:
* The academic assessor is or may be the personal tutor for the student that they are confirming, but not for concurrent parts of the programme. For example, for a 3-year programme, the academic assessor is assigned for parts 1 and 3 or for one part of the programme only. Part is defined as each year of the programme.
* For a 2-year programme, a different academic assessor will be assigned for each part of the programme.

- The academic assessor may remain the student's personal tutor for the duration of the programme.
- The NMC is clear that practice assessors are not simultaneously the practice supervisor and academic assessor for the same student, and practice assessors for students on NMC-approved prescribing programmes support learning in line with the NMC standards for prescribing programmes.

The NMC (2018c) in *Part 2: Standards for student supervision and assessment* is clear that the academic assessor should be aware of any concerns regarding student performance, including any concerns that may have been raised in the practice environment or by practice assessors. The NMC provides information on its website around this topic, as summarised below:

- The academic assessor may have a role in improving the student's performance and this includes developing an action plan in partnership with the student.
- The academic assessor role will depend on several different factors, such as the student's stage of learning and the academic assessor's involvement in it, and any policies or procedures within their university for improving student performance.
- If the student is not meeting required actions, the academic assessor should take any appropriate action, which may include recommending the student be failed on that part of the programme, or that they do not progress. This should be done through discussion with the nominated practice assessor, following any academic processes set in place by the university and their practice learning partners.
- If there is an immediate concern or risk to the public from the student's performance the academic assessor must take appropriate action, such as recommending the student for removal or suspension from a learning environment or course. This should be done through following university fitness to practise policy and should involve the practice assessor.
- Students with disabilities are entitled to have reasonable adjustments considered in relation to their practice learning. However, while reasonable adjustments may be made to the way that a student meets a competency or standard, the competency or standard itself cannot be adjusted.

Figure 2.1 presented later in this chapter provides an example of processes for dealing with any concerns or disagreements in relation to students' learning and development, demonstrating that this will be a team approach involving, for example, the practice assessor and practice education facilitator.

Academic assessors tend to work in higher education institutions, but some individuals may work in roles that span both university and practice settings. Practice supervisors and assessors will need to work closely with academic assessors, so it is important for everyone to have an awareness of each other's roles and responsibilities.

☑ ACTIVITY 2.9

Familiarise yourself with the local arrangements for communication between practice supervisors, assessors and academic assessors. As a practice assessor, what information will you be required to gather in readiness for your meetings about the learners in your area?

This is a personal reflective activity, so no answer guide is provided.

Table 2.5 identifies the knowledge, skills and behaviours and role preparation required by the academic assessor.

Role preparation and ongoing support in the role for academic assessors can take several different forms, such as access to student documentation, knowing what the student is expected to achieve, protected time to attend training, and support for raising concerns. It can also involve access to student learning records in practice or even physical access to different learning environments. They should also have the protected time to carry out their role, including time for completing any student records.

While support is proportionate it will depend on the individual academic assessor and what is needed for them to perform their role and uphold public protection. Regardless, all academic assessors should have access to a range of teaching resources and updates, both online and taught, to enable continuing skills and knowledge development for their job role. They should also be provided with resources to access, reading and updates relevant to their needs.

Table 2.6 provides examples of development opportunities that can help you to prepare and maintain your knowledge, skills and behaviours. It will be useful for you to find out how you will demonstrate to your organisation that you have met and are maintaining proficiency in the role.

Table 2.5: *Academic assessor role preparation*

Knowledge	Skills	Behaviours
Demonstrate and maintain current knowledge and expertise relevant for the proficiencies and programme outcomes they are assessing and confirming	Collate and confirm student achievement of proficiencies and programme outcomes in the academic environment for each part of the programme	Role model behaviours demonstrating that they are receiving ongoing support and training to reflect and develop in their role
Understand the student's learning and achievement in practice	Make and record objective, evidence-based decisions on conduct, proficiency and achievement, and recommendations for progression, drawing on student records and other resources; conduct objective, evidence-based assessments of students	Apply leadership skills through proactively developing their professional practice and knowledge in order to fulfil their role
Understand the proficiencies and programme outcomes that the student they confirm is aiming to achieve	Partnership working with a nominated practice assessor to evaluate and recommend the student for progression for each part of the programme, in line with programme standards and local and national policies	
Knowledge of the assessment process and their role within it (preparation)	Time management and communication skills to communicate, collaborate and manage student progression with practice assessors at scheduled and relevant points in programme structure	
Understand the proficiencies and programme outcomes that the student they assess is aiming to achieve	Demonstrate interpersonal communication skills, relevant to student learning and assessment (preparation)	
	Provide constructive feedback to facilitate professional development in others	

Table 2.6: Example of development opportunities to help prepare and maintain academic assessor knowledge, skills and behaviours

Knowledge	Skills	Behaviours
Read and become familiar with the NMC standards for student supervision and assessment	Workshop attendance (face-to-face or online)	Use reflection to examine your own practice and ongoing development, using revalidation and personal development review to support the process
Find out about proficiencies and programme outcomes you are supporting students to achieve, from the university and NMC website	Simulation-based education	Consider use of testimonies from others to understand your communication skills and partnership working with other members of the education team, particularly the practice assessor
	Undertake a preparation programme developed collaboratively between the university and practice partner healthcare organisations, focusing on the role core skills such as assessment and feedback	Identify who will support and guide you in your role and how this support will be accessed, focusing on areas such as resilience and how you respond to difficult situations around challenging assessment, underperforming students and raising concerns; particularly how you communicate with the practice assessor and other members of the education team
	Undertake professional development activities, utilising relevant educational resources such as effective application of policies and procedures when collating and confirming student progression	

Universities also need to develop models so that the academic assessor is clear on how students progress through a programme of study. Below is an example of a pre-registration nursing programme progression chart (*Table 2.7*) for a 3-year undergraduate programme, in which the student undertakes three practice experiences (placements) per year. Demonstrated is where the communication takes place between the practice and academic assessor and points in the programme where students can retrieve proficiencies not previously achieved within the part of the programme. For this example, the 'part' equates to each year of the programme.

The progression chart acknowledges NMC requirements for registration such as students engaging with medicines management, episodes of care assessment, assessment of proficiencies and professional values.

Table 2.7: Pre-registration nursing programme progression chart (3-year duration)

Programme timing	Academic assessor/personal tutor role requirement
1. During practice learning experience (all parts)	If there are any concerns at the start of or during placement, the AA will work with the PA to devise and complete an action plan that is recorded in PARE AA/PT meetings as identified in PARE document and negotiated with the student where concerns are raised, or support required Student made aware of pastoral, health and wellbeing support via Student HuB
2. End of part/ placement review during practice learning experience three	AA will have scheduled communication and collaboration with PA via mutually agreed mode, e.g. Skype, and the record will be completed utilising the record of communication page in PARE by the identified submission date If there are any concerns, the AA will work with the PA to devise and complete an action plan that is recorded in PARE Students should have completed the professional values for this practice learning experience, all the proficiencies, episode of care both formative and summative and medicines management; in addition, for all students, the OAR should be completed in collaboration with the PA and PS. The AA should monitor the students' hours of progress at regular intervals on the programme to ensure a timely completion, ensuring students complete 37.5 hours per week especially when undertaking long days to minimise a deficit at the end of the allocated placement; any concerns re hours should then be escalated to the PL if not resolvable by the PT
3. Preparation for board of examiner progression meeting	AA to confirm to PL by a set date (date communicated by the PL) that the proficiencies for the programme/part are verified PL reports to and confirms at the assessment board
4. Board of examiner requirements	PL presents the results to the assessment board and at this point, where the student is progressed, then there will be the rotation of the AA role
5. Retrieval of practice competencies/ proficiencies	AA and PA to work collaboratively to devise an action plan to support the student through the retrieval period, clearly identifying the proficiencies to be achieved OAR retrieval to be completed by set retrieval date by AA and PA; report and record at board of examiner progression meeting AA roles as in steps 1 and 2 Students: professional values for trimester 3 will be considered as both a first attempt at this board and if required as a reassessment
6. End of programme/ part 3	During this time students should be virtually meeting weekly with their PA/PS for 1 hour per week (recorded on the progressions towards registration page) AA weekly review of documentation where concerns are raised, with follow-up actions with PA In conjunction with the PA and AA, there will be a review of the whole assessment documentation including student reflections; check that the PA has confirmed the student is practising independently with minimal supervision and has achieved all the requirements of final part

Table 2.7: *(cont'd)*

Programme timing	Academic assessor/personal tutor role requirement
	The OAR is completed by the AA who informs the programme lead in time for the assessment board, date relayed by the PL. For unsuccessful students the retrieval process is as above (see point 5). The AA will confirm the retrieval outcome to inform the PL in time for the final progression assessment board.
7. Programme and NMC requirements	PL checks that student has met programme and NMC requirements (i.e. met programme hours), liaising with personal tutor around the personal circumstances of the student Student is required to complete good health and character page via PARE Administration upload student details to NMC portal PL makes decision about health and character of students via the NMC portal Student receives PIN number

AA, *academic assessor;* OAR, *ongoing achievement record;* PA, *practice assessor;* PARE, *practice assessment record and evaluation;* PL, *programme leader;* PS, *practice supervisor;* PT, *personal tutor.*

2.5.4 The wider education team: the practice education facilitator

What is becoming clear is the range of people who will be working as supervisor and assessors, all of whom contribute to the decision-making process around student progression through the programme and ultimately NMC registration. Often supervisors and assessors are required to juggle the increasing demands of delivering patient care alongside their supervisory or assessor roles. In order to support the process of learning and assessing in clinical practice, some organisations may identify specific individuals who have a clinical education remit, whose role it is to support supervisors and assessors. These specific individuals may include the **practice education facilitator** or **clinical educator**, with titles varying from within and across healthcare organisations. For further information about the practice educator role see the paper by Maxwell *et al.* (2015) in *Recommended further reading.*

Noticeable within the mentorship supervisory model is the team approach whereby a team of supervisors support students in clinical practice. Influenced by evidence from the 2012 Willis Commission on the future of nursing education, there is an increased emphasis on models of support that adopt coaching approaches to student clinical development, the coaching model advocated by Willis being the Collaborative Learning in Practice model (CLiP) (Willis, 2015). Coaching models that promote the development of nursing students' clinical leadership often utilise peer learning and are perfect for the new NMC standards, which require students to take responsibility for their own knowledge acquisition (Leigh and Littlewood, 2018). In *Chapter 3* the GM Synergy model is introduced; it demonstrates how the NMC supervisor and assessor roles complement a coaching approach to student learning and development and promote clinical leadership development.

The clinical educator role, for example, is fundamental to the success of the CLiP model. For further information about this model of supporting student learning you might want to see the following paper presented at a conference about the project by Lobo *et al.* (2014): www.charleneloboconsulting.com/wp-content/uploads/CLiP-Paper-final-version-Sept-14.pdf

2.6 MANAGING DISAGREEMENT ABOUT STUDENT PROGRESSION

The NMC is clear that no student should progress through a course or enter the register when they are not fit to do so. The university, in partnership with its practice learning partners, is responsible for putting in place the right processes to ensure this does not happen. There is useful information on the NMC website to support your understanding and actions to be taken.

Universities, together with practice learning partners, should have in place mechanisms for managing disagreement about student progression; for example through appeals or complaints. This includes disagreements between practice and academic assessors and disagreements from the students. Discussed earlier in the chapter is the role of the academic assessor.

Examples of potential disagreements include the initial, mid-term and final assessments not carried out at appropriate time points, or disagreements around appropriate support for the student in practice by the practice assessor, supervisor or academic assessor. Another example is where the student's attendance in practice is questioned. Where due process has not been followed, disagreements should only relate to process and not assessment.

Figure 2.1 is an example of a flowchart for dealing with any concerns or disagreements in relation to students' learning and development. Notice the involvement of the wider practice learning team who have a role in responding to and managing concerns and disagreements; for example, the practice education facilitator.

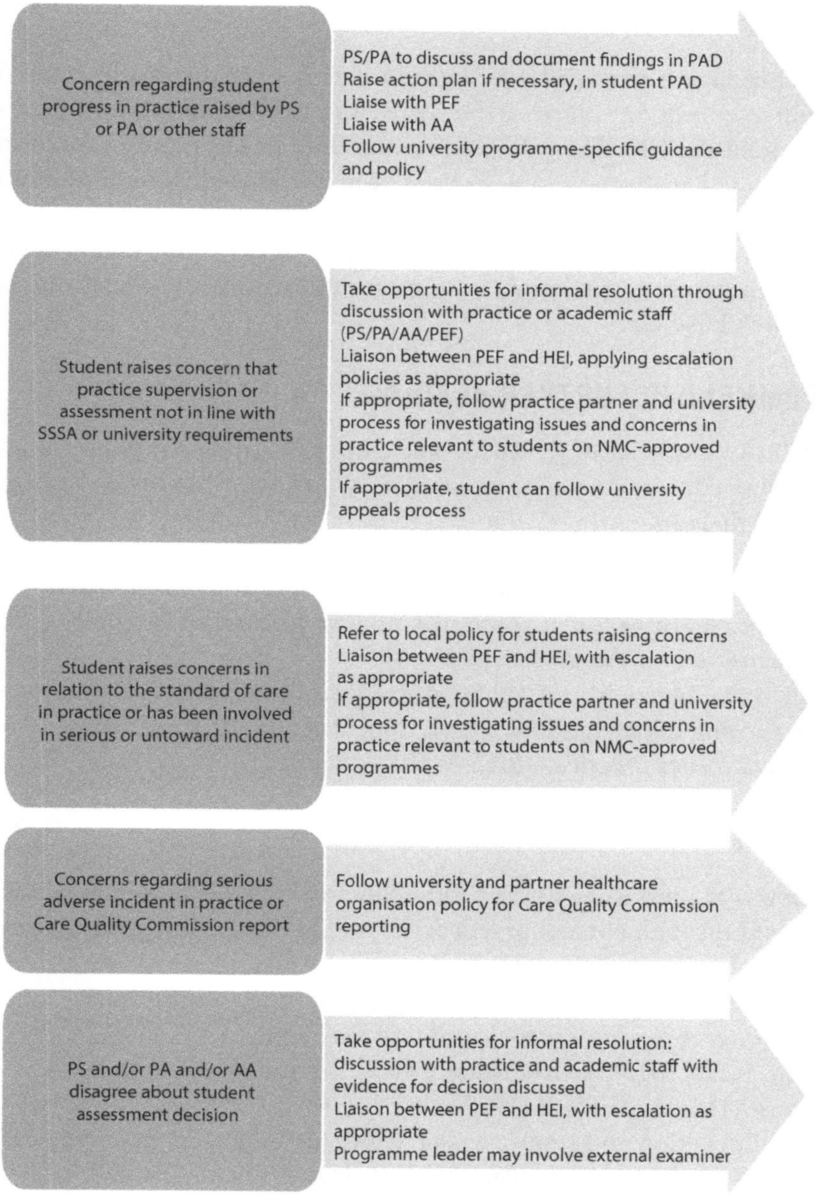

Figure 2.1: *Overview of processes for dealing with any concerns or disagreements in relation to students' learning and development.*
AA, academic assessor; PA, practice assessor; PAD, practice assessment document; PEF, practice education facilitator; PS, practice supervisor; SSSA, Part 2: Standards for student supervision and assessment (NMC, 2018c).

2.7 SUMMARY

This chapter has provided you with an overview of the global standards for nurse education and then presented the new standards in operation throughout the UK. The roles and responsibilities of practice supervisors, assessors and academic assessors have been introduced. After undertaking the activities and reading the recommended papers you should now have a better understanding of these new roles and how you might develop your own practice in relation to supporting learning, in order to make it everyone's business.

RECOMMENDED FURTHER READING

Flott, E.A. and Linden, L. (2016) The clinical learning environment in nursing education: a concept analysis. *Journal of Advanced Nursing*, **72(3)**: 501–13.

Maxwell, E., Black, S. and Baillie, L. (2015) The role of the practice educator in supporting nursing and midwifery students' clinical practice learning: an appreciative inquiry. *Journal of Nursing Education and Practice*, **5(1)**: 35–45.

Tee, S. and Cowen, M. (2012) Supporting students with disabilities – promoting understanding amongst mentors in practice. *Nurse Education in Practice*, **12(1)**: 6–10.

REFERENCES

Andrews, M. and Roberts, D. (2003) Supporting student nurses learning in and through clinical practice: the role of the clinical guide. *Nurse Education Today*, **23**: 471–81.

Cranton, P. (2016) *Understanding and promoting transformative learning: A guide to theory and practice*. Stylus.

Dalton, N.S. (2013) Neurodiversity HCI. *Interactions*. **20(2)**: 72–5. doi:10.1145/2427076.2427091

Health Education and Improvement Wales (2018) *Practice supervisor/ practice assessor guide: Part 2: NMC standards for student supervision and assessment* (2018). HEIW. Available at: https://heiw. nhs.wales/files/once-for-wales-docs/all-wales-practice-supervisor-assessor-guide/ (accessed 13 August 2020).

Helminen, K., Coco, K., Johnson, M., Turunen, H. and Tossavainen, K. (2016) Summative assessment of clinical practice of student nurses: A review of the literature. *International Journal of Nursing Studies*, **53**: 308–19.

Henderson, A. and Eaton, E. (2013) Assisting nurses to facilitate student and new graduate learning in practice settings: What 'support' do nurses at the bedside need? *Nurse Education in Practice*, **13**: 197–201.

Leigh, J.A. and Littlewood, L. (2018) Providing the right environment to develop new clinical nurse leaders. *British Journal of Nursing*, **27(6)**: 341–3. doi: 10.12968/bjon.2018.27.6.341

Lobo, C., Arthur, A. and Latimer, V. (2014) *Collaborative Learning in Practice (CLiP) for pre-registration nursing students.* University of East Anglia. Available at: www.charleneloboconsulting.com/wp-content/uploads/CLiP-Paper-final-version-Sept-14.pdf (accessed 13 August 2020).

Nursing and Midwifery Council (2010) *Standards for pre-registration nurse education.* NMC. Available at: www.nmc.org.uk/globalassets/sitedocuments/standards/nmc-standards-for-pre-registration-nursing-education.pdf (accessed 13 August 2020).

Nursing and Midwifery Council (2018a) *Future nurse: Standards of proficiency for registered nurses.* London: NMC. Available at: www.nmc.org.uk/globalassets/sitedocuments/education-standards/future-nurse-proficiencies.pdf (accessed 13 August 2020).

Nursing and Midwifery Council (2018b) *Realising professionalism: Part 1: Standards framework for nursing and midwifery education.* NMC. Available at: www.nmc.org.uk/globalassets/sitedocuments/education-standards/education-framework.pdf (accessed 13 August 2020).

Nursing and Midwifery Council (2018c) *Realising professionalism: Part 2: Standards for student supervision and assessment.* NMC. Available at: www.nmc.org.uk/globalassets/sitedocuments/education-standards/student-supervision-assessment.pdf (accessed 13 August 2020).

Nursing and Midwifery Council (2018d) *Realising professionalism: Part 3: Standards for education and training.* NMC. Available at: www.nmc.org.uk/globalassets/sitedocuments/education-standards/programme-standards-nursing.pdf (accessed 13 August 2020).

Nursing and Midwifery Council (2018e) *The Code: Professional standards of practice and behaviour for nurses, midwives and nursing associates.* NMC. Available at: www.nmc.org.uk/globalassets/sitedocuments/nmc-publications/nmc-code.pdf (accessed 29 September 2020).

Pitkänen, S., Kääriäinen, M., Oikarainen, A. *et al.* (2018) Healthcare students' evaluation of the clinical learning environment and supervision – a cross-sectional study. *Nurse Education Today*, **62**: 143–9.

Roberts, D. (2011) Grading the performance of clinical skills: Lessons to be learned from the performing arts. *Nurse Education Today*, **31**: 607–10.

Royal College of Nursing Wales (2016) *The future of nursing education in Wales*. RCN Wales. Available at: www.rcn.org.uk/about-us/our-influencing-work/policy-briefings/education-strategy (accessed 30 November 2020).

Royal College of Nursing (2017) *Helping students get the best from their practice placements: A Royal College of Nursing toolkit*. RCN. Available at: https://scadmin.rcn.org.uk/-/media/royal-college-of-nursing/documents/publications/2017/may/pub-006035.pdf (accessed 30 November 2020).

Wainwright, T.W., McDonald, D.A. and Burgess, L.C. (2017) The role of physiotherapy in enhanced recovery after surgery in the intensive care unit. *ICU Management and Practice*, **17**(3): 144–7. Available at: https://healthmanagement.org/uploads/article_attachment/icu-v17-i3-wainwright-physiotherapyineras.pdf (accessed 13 August 2020).

Willis G.P. (2015) *Shape of caring: A review of the future education and training of registered nurses and care assistants*. Health Education England. Available at: www.hee.nhs.uk/sites/default/files/documents/2348-Shape-of-caring-review-FINAL.pdf (accessed 13 August 2020).

World Health Organization (2009) *Global standards for the initial education of professional nurses and midwives*. WHO. Available at: www.who.int/hrh/nursing_midwifery/hrh_global_standards_education.pdf (accessed 13 August 2020).

World Health Organization (2020) *State of the world's nursing 2020*. WHO. Available at: www.who.int/publications/i/item/9789240003279 (accessed 30 November 2020).

ACTIVITY ANSWER GUIDE

ACTIVITY 2.4

	Related to the patient	Related to the student
Knowledge	Anatomy and physiology of the chest Abnormal breath sounds	Academic level of the programme the student is studying Recognition of prior learning Appropriate range of clinical teaching techniques
Skills	Communication skills (age appropriate), including use of therapeutic touch Location of physical landmarks and chest auscultation Applying suction to remove secretions if required	Communication skills Demonstration skills
Attitudes	Person-centred or holistic care	Impact of self as a role model for the student Open interprofessional learning

USING COACHING CONVERSATIONS AND COACHING MODELS TO PROMOTE EFFECTIVE SUPERVISION AND ASSESSMENT

Jacqueline Leigh, Kisma Anderson, Anne Medcalf, Andrea Surtees and Wendy Sutton

3.1 INTRODUCTION

According to the Nursing and Midwifery Council (NMC) standards for education and training *Part 2: Standards for student supervision and assessment*:

> "*Students in practice or work-placed learning must be supported to learn. This may include being supernumerary, meaning that they are not counted as part of the staffing required for safe and effective care in that setting. The decision on the level of supervision provided for students should be based on the needs of the individual student. The level of supervision can decrease with the student's increasing proficiency and confidence. Students must be provided with adjustments in accordance with relevant equalities and human rights legislation in all learning environments and for supervision and assessment*".
> (NMC, 2018b, p. 4)

Part 2 of the NMC standards can be accessed here:
www.nmc.org.uk/globalassets/sitedocuments/education-standards/student-supervision-assessment.pdf

This chapter focuses on mechanisms that can be used in clinical practice by supervisors and assessors to support student learning through coaching. The new standards emphasise the need for students to be supported towards independent learning. The use of coaching as a mechanism to support learning can help practice supervisors from a range of disciplines and professions to fulfil the requirements of the role in terms of support and feedback.

Coaching is an intervention that facilitates another person's learning, development and performance. Applied to student learning in practice, coaching has the potential to promote effective supervision and assessment and to support clinical leadership development. Coaching is student led, less focused on following the directions of a clinical supervisor and more focused on students taking responsibility for identifying their learning goals and objectives: hence working towards becoming independent learners and eventually independent nurses (Leigh *et al.*, 2019).

This chapter defines and explores the nature of coaching as applied to supporting learning in practice. By the end of the chapter you will have a better practical understanding of the differences between coaching and mentoring. Through engaging in a series of activities, you will examine the core concepts of coaching conversations that when applied to supervision and assessment of students, effectively facilitate student learning. The qualities of the effective coach in clinical practice are explored and, through the use of a case study, you will apply a coaching model in clinical practice that sets out coach–student expectations and promotes student wellbeing.

After reading this chapter you will be able to:

- Define coaching
- Explore the similarities and differences between coaching and mentoring
- Explore how coaching conversations can facilitate effective supervision and assessment in clinical practice and clinical leadership development
- Understand the qualities of the effective coach in clinical practice
- Using the Greater Manchester (GM) Synergy model as an example, apply a coaching model in clinical practice that sets out coach–student expectations and facilitates student learning, clinical leadership development and promotes wellbeing.

3.2 COACHING AND MENTORING

Coaching can be defined in many ways that includes unlocking a person's potential to maximise their performance (Whitmore, 2017). The *Cambridge Dictionary* defines coaching as "the act of giving special classes in sports, a school subject, or a work-related activity, especially to one person or a small group" (*Cambridge Dictionary*, https://dictionary.cambridge.org/).

In relation to students, unlocking a student's potential suggests that coaching is an action or change-orientated process that requires someone to work in partnership with the student to help them make the change and help with setting the direction that they choose to take. For the purpose of this chapter, coaching is defined as an approach adopted by supervisors and assessors that facilitates the students learning and development, and this is achieved through unlocking the student's own potential. As such, it is a strengths-based approach and this is reflected in the skills required by the proficiencies outlined in Annexe A of *Future nurse: Standards of proficiency for registered nurses* (NMC, 2018a).

Mentoring on the other hand is traditionally more concerned with providing advice, guidance and opinion and is based on a relationship whereby the mentor uses their knowledge and wisdom to provide advice that is based on what experience has taught them. The Royal College of Nursing (RCN) in their *Guidance for mentors of nursing and midwifery students* (RCN, 2017) clearly identifies that as well as providing support and guidance to students in the practice area, mentors have the unique opportunity to role model the professional values and behaviours and to instil professional integrity. This includes professional socialisation and the promotion of positive values, attitudes, behaviours, cultural variances and inclusivity.

In reality there is an overlap of features between coaching and mentoring and it is useful to think about the words of John Whitmore (2017) who states that whether we coach, advise, counsel, facilitate or mentor, the effectiveness of what we do depends in large measure on our beliefs about human potential and that the person has the capability to make any changes that can positively affect what they do.

For Whitmore therefore, coaching delivers in large measure because of the supportive relationship between the coach and the coachee, and means and style of communication used. In relation to the role of the practice supervisor, practice assessor and academic assessor, taking on a coaching approach requires the building of a relationship that is underpinned by effective communication. It could be argued that the principles of coaching or mentoring will be evident within all three of the new roles outlined by the NMC (2018b) to some extent, although they may manifest in different ways. For example, as you work through this chapter you will see that the practice assessor when assessing student proficiency can use the core concepts of coaching conversations such as active listening, effective questioning and feedback.

ACTIVITY 3.1

Based on your values and beliefs, construct your own definition of coaching or add to the above definition. Write your definition down as you will refer to it throughout this chapter.

This is a personal reflective activity, so no answer guide is provided.

3.3 PROMOTING EFFECTIVE SUPERVISION, ASSESSMENT AND CLINICAL LEADERSHIP DEVELOPMENT THROUGH COACHING IN CLINICAL PRACTICE

Adopting a coaching style in supervision and assessment provides students with the opportunity to take responsibility for their own knowledge acquisition. For example, the role of the practice supervisor as set out in the Part 2 NMC (2018b) standards is to:

- role model and facilitate learning of students through independent participation
- raise and respond to competency and conduct concerns
- supervise, support and provide feedback to students
- contribute to assessment and progress decisions made by assessors.

This in turn promotes optimal patient care, achieved through improved student performance, motivation and empowerment. There is also a positive impact on developing the student's clinical leadership skills.

Table 3.1 summarises the differences between coaching and mentoring in the context of supervision and assessment.

Table 3.1: Differences between coaching and mentoring in the context of supervision and assessment

Mentoring	Coaching
Answers questions	Asks questions
Steps in and provides care	Steps back and allows the student to learn by providing care
Is watched by the student	Watches the student
Directs the student's learning	The student demonstrates what they have learnt (usually self-directed) to the coach
Allocates work to the student	Is allocated work by the student
Talks	Listens
Does the same work as before	Works differently, while coaching the student
Identifies individual learning opportunities in the whole practice learning environment	Uses the whole practice learning area as a complete learning environment

Student nurses often experience pressures outside of their academic/ placement life. Nursing students are said to have increased stress due to competing demands and challenges of nurse education (Watson *et al.*, 2017). Indeed, McCarthy *et al.* (2018, p. 197) go so far as to say that "stress is pervasive in all aspects of undergraduate nursing and midwifery education".

There is a requirement therefore for supervisors and assessors to be proficient in the skills of coaching conversations so that they can effectively identify and manage the student's learning and pastoral needs, and this is achieved through unlocking the student's potential for learning and development. Through coaching, supervisors and assessors can get the best out of their students through balancing the following three needs:

1. The needs of the student (learning/pastoral)
2. The needs of the university (delivering on the high-quality student experience), and
3. The needs of the practice placement areas (to deliver high-quality patient care).

ACTIVITY 3.2

Write down the benefits and risks of adopting a coaching approach to student supervision and assessment. Once you have done this, consider strategies to reduce the identified risks.

An answer guide is provided at the end of the chapter.

You may have identified a benefit that focuses on how coaching can promote leadership learning that is student led, less focused on following the directions of a practice supervisor and more focused on students taking responsibility for identifying their learning goals and objectives.

Risks may include, for example, a student's readiness for their increased responsibility and the coach in clinical practice feeling prepared and adequately supported in their role to enable the student to fulfil those increased responsibilities. Effective communication across the entire team is crucial in ensuring that everyone is aware of their role in student learning. This awareness is one way of reducing risk.

Next, through engaging in a series of activities, you will examine the core concepts of coaching conversations that, when applied to supervision and assessment of students, effectively facilitate student learning.

3.4 EXPLORING THE CORE CONCEPTS OF COACHING CONVERSATIONS

Coaching conversations are the lynchpin to effective communication with students in clinical practice by helping students to focus their thinking about their learning. This can be achieved through effective questioning, active listening and by providing feedback (feedback is explored further in

Chapter 5 of this book). The first core concept to be explored is effective questioning.

3.4.1 *Effective questioning*

During clinical placement students will have NMC proficiencies they need to develop, skills they need to cultivate and goals they want to achieve. While they may be clear about what they need, the reality of how to go about achieving them in the context of a specific learning environment may be more challenging. Effective questioning skills on the part of the supervisor can empower the student to generate more relevant thinking around such challenges and develop their problem-solving skills. It should be remembered, however, that enabling the student to do this requires great skill. Questioning at:

> *"too low or high a level will not increase learning; too low: nothing new will be learned, and too high: will go over the student's head. Those teaching students in practice settings must understand this concept; the real skill is to outline new information in such a way that allows the student's existing understanding to assimilate the new knowledge into their cognitive structures"*. (Andrews and Roberts, 2003, p. 477)

Socratic questioning, for example, is the disciplined practice of thoughtful questioning which enables the student to examine ideas logically to determine the validity of those ideas and to explore ideas in depth. According to Straker (2010), the overall purpose of Socratic questioning is to challenge accuracy and completeness of thinking in a way that acts to move people towards their ultimate goal. Practice supervisors using Socratic questioning promote person-centred learning, enhance problem-solving capabilities in the student and help the student construct their knowledge base.

Examples of Socratic questions used by practice supervisors are offered in *Table 3.2*.

Table 3.2: Socratic questions used by practice supervisors

Type of question	Example of use
Questions for clarification	What is your rationale for choosing that dressing? How does this relate to our discussion about achieving your proficiencies?
Questions that probe assumptions	What could we assume about the client's choice of dress instead? How can you verify or refute that assumption? Why are we not challenging the multidisciplinary team over Mr Ahmed's package of care?

Table 3.2: (cont'd)

Type of question	Example of use
Questions that probe reasons and evidence	What do you think caused Mrs Jones's blood pressure to drop? Do you think that having the sink positioned in the corner of the ward has increased handwashing and decreased infection rates, therefore worth the cost to install?
Questions about viewpoints and perspectives	Are there alternative pressure-relieving devices that could be used by Mr Read in this situation? What is another viewpoint about person-centred care?
Questions that probe implications and consequences	What are the consequences of that assumption made about Isabelle's nutrition plan? What are you implying?

Practice assessors can also apply Socratic questioning to inform the robust and objective assessment decision-making process, with *Table 3.3* providing examples that could be applied.

Table 3.3: Socratic questions used by the practice assessor

Type of question	Example of use
Questions for clarification	What is your rationale for choosing that dressing?
Questions that probe assumptions	Tell me about the client's choice of dress? Tell me why you have not challenged the multidisciplinary team over Mr Ahmed's package of care?
Questions that probe reasons and evidence	What do you think caused Mrs Jones's blood pressure to drop? Can you explain how you will apply the sepsis protocol with Mrs Jones?
Questions about viewpoints and perspectives	What alternative pressure-relieving devices did you consider for Mr Read? Tell me about your definition of person-centred care and how you have applied it to managing patient care on the surgical ward?
Questions that probe implications and consequences	What is the impact of your decision-making on Isabelle's nutrition plan?

For further information about the background to Socratic questioning you might want to access Dinkins and Cangelosi (2019) from *Recommended further reading.*

✎ **ACTIVITY 3.3**

Consider the following two statements offered by John Whitmore (2017, p. 81) who explores the use of different questioning approaches when holding coaching conversations. Decide if you agree or disagree with the statements.
1. Telling or asking closed questions saves people from having to think.
2. Asking open questions causes individuals to think for themselves (Whitmore, 2017).

Based on your definition of coaching, which type of questioning would best unlock the student's potential for learning?
    The answer to this activity is outlined as you progress through this section of the chapter.

Drawing on your response to *Activity 3.3*, you may have considered that the practice supervisor, through asking open questions (questions that cannot be answered with a yes or no response) generates thinking in the student and invites them to give more in-depth responses. This in turn enables the practice supervisor to review the student's knowledge and understanding around a skill or task. It also provides insight to the practice supervisor about the student's thinking around their goals or challenges and their readiness for formal assessment. In other words, and according to Kline (2015), incisive questions can challenge assumptions in the coachee's (student's) thinking process and lead to 'light bulb' moments.

   Open questions generally start with a who, what, when, where or how? They are used to elicit information about thoughts, knowledge, feelings and opinions. These may be used for example at the start of a discussion with a student about a skill they wish to develop, for example in *Scenario 3.1*.

📁 **SCENARIO 3.1**

Practice supervisor: "Good morning Lucy, following handover this morning you identified that you would like to undertake some of the wound care procedures today. What other practice learning experiences have you had with wound care?"
    Holding the conversation with the coach using closed questions generates a very different response, for example:
    Practice supervisor: "Good morning Lucy, following handover this morning you identified that you would like to undertake some of the wound care procedures today. Have you done wound care before?"
    As the open question discussion proceeds, the student may tell you about caring for a person with a wound that they have experienced before.

> 🏳 **SCENARIO 3.1** *(cont'd)*
>
> Combining a probing question with the open question not only enables the practice supervisor to find out more detail about the student's experiences but also demonstrates their interest in what the student has to say. Indeed, demonstrating interest is critical in developing the coaching relationship.
>
> Practice supervisor: "That's interesting; tell me more about how you dealt with this kind of wound?"
>
> The practice supervisor, using the combination of coaching questions, provides the student with the opportunity to elaborate on their experiences by providing more detail during which they may tell you about a specific wound dressing used and some of the challenges experienced during a dressing change. Again, to elicit more detail the coach would follow up with a focused question.
>
> Practice supervisor: "That must have been a difficult situation Lucy, what actions did you take?"
>
> By applying the range of questioning techniques such as open, focused and probing questions and avoiding closed questions, the practice supervisor has enabled the student to reflect on their own experiences and demonstrate their knowledge and understanding. The practice supervisor at the same time has been able to make judgements about the student's skills and abilities, thus determining the level of supervision required, i.e. either direct or indirect supervision or delegation.

The types of questions that promote effective coaching conversations are summarised in *Table 3.4*.

Table 3.4: Types of questions that promote effective coaching conversations

Type of question	Example of use
Open: to promote the discussion (What, Where, When, How, Why need to be used carefully to avoid appearing judgemental)	Tell me about your experiences with ….
Probing: to follow up on what has been said	What were your feelings at the time? What action will you take?
Focused: to establish the real situation and real actions to be taken	What were your feelings at the time? What actions will you take?

Types of questions to be avoided are leading questions. This is because this type of questioning would subtly prompt the student to answer in a certain way. An example of a leading question is: "You do not always choose the same type of dressing for Mr Lee's leg ulcer, do you?".

An alternative question using the open question would be: "Tell me about the range of dressings that could be used on Mr Lee's leg ulcer?".

Types of questions to be used selectively are closed questions. This is because this type of question produces the single word or short phrase response, and thus does not encourage open discussion. For example: "Do you know what time Mrs Brown takes her insulin?".

☑ ACTIVITY 3.4

It would be useful to reflect on a situation where you have held a conversation with a student about progress in meeting their NMC programme proficiencies. Write down the types of questions that you used and consider their effectiveness. Consider a different questioning technique and write down the benefits that this could have when making decisions about a student's progress and building the coaching relationship and in determining the level of supervision required.

This is a personal reflective activity, so no answer guide is provided.

The second coaching concept to be explored is active listening.

3.4.2 Active listening

It may be useful to consider that there are different levels of active listening. For the purpose of this chapter, *Figure 3.1* identifies three levels and as you progress through this section of the chapter, consider what are your personal actions to advance towards demonstrating Level 3 Global listening skills.

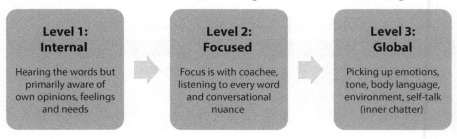

Figure 3.1: *Levels of listening (adapted from Kimsey-House et al., 2011).*

A crucial element of coaching conversations is active listening. Coaching conversations should be led by the student, and what they are saying should be the focal point. Allowing students time to think and respond to questions during the conversation enables them to really consider their goals or challenges. Actively listening and paying attention to someone when they are talking has a powerful effect. The speaker feels like they matter, that their words have value, that their contribution is important, that perhaps they can speak freely and openly. Actively listening (listening without judging or interrupting) improves the individual's thinking (Kline, 2015).

ACTIVITY 3.5

Think about the last time someone listened to you in this way (actively listened). How did it make you feel?

Now think about the last time you tried to speak to someone who did not provide their undivided attention; perhaps they were called away mid-sentence or they stopped to take a call. How did that make you feel?

This is a personal reflective activity, so no answer guide is provided.

Active listening, as its name suggests, is not a passive activity and indeed takes practice to perfect. When developing our active listening skills, we need to consider our own internal chatter. Internal chatter is an introspective monitoring or self-governing of our feelings which provides the checks and balances on our actions throughout the day. It is this dialogue that can drive self-reflection and motivation but also self-criticism and thus self-doubt (and often keeps us awake at night). Active listening requires the listener to 'quiet' this chatter and focus on the speaker and what they are saying. This is different to not simply thinking of your next coaching question or inserting yourself into their dialogue, providing examples of what you would do in a certain situation or instructing them on what they should do with your own 'expert advice'. That is not to say that we are not experienced professionals in our own right or that at times the student may simply need advice or instruction, rather that coaching conversations are about truly listening to what the speaker (student) has to say, and through incisive questioning on the part of the coach unlocking the student's potential and having belief in their ability to problem solve and find solutions to their own challenges and goals.

"It is questions rather than instructions or advice that best generate awareness and responsibility." (Whitmore, 2017, p. 81)

ACTIVITY 3.6

How do you demonstrate that you are listening and have heard what has been said?

An answer guide is provided at the end of the chapter.

For the practice supervisor, active listening will be a crucial skill to develop. This is because the practice supervisor is the healthcare professional who will spend most of the time on placement with the student, assisting them to meet their NMC proficiencies and individual practice learning goals. The practice supervisor role is discussed in detail in *Chapter 1*. The first opportunity to truly practise active listening will be during the initial meeting when the student commences their practice placement where the student will talk about their self-assessment and identify what they want to achieve. Practice learning goals should be set by the student themselves, with the supervisor actively listening as they talk about how they will go about formulating and achieving these. Through open questioning and active listening the practice supervisor can facilitate the student in developing a meaningful action plan for their clinical placement.

3.4.3 Giving feedback

Giving feedback is the third and final core concept to be explored in this chapter. This is expanded on more fully in *Chapter 5*.

Giving constructive feedback is a critical component in teaching, assessing and supervising students. It can range from something as simple as an encouraging observation to a more structured written statement in the student's practise assessment document (usually following verbal discussion). It is such a powerful tool that has potential to accelerate a student's learning but if done poorly or without due care and attention can be destructive to the student–supervisor relationship, to the student's confidence and, if not done at all, can result in unchecked poor and even unsafe practice potentially putting patients at risk.

Sadly, feedback can often be associated with criticism both by the person providing the feedback, hence their reluctance to give it, and by the person receiving it which can result in angry retaliations or tears, particularly if feedback is in relation to 'failing' or poor performance (Duffy, 2013). This has led to a shift away from the term constructive criticism due to the negative connotations of the word 'criticism' to terms such as constructive feedback.

Feedback which is not targeted, planned or personalised can fall short of its intended purpose and is ineffective in terms of helping the student to have insights about their behaviour or thinking/problem-solving processes (Clynes and Raftery, 2008; Starr, 2016). Constructive feedback on the other hand is honest and sincere and when given with positive intention based on facts and not assumptions, can inspire and motivate students, helping them to feel valued. To do this effectively requires trust between practice supervisor and student in the supervisory relationship.

In her work '*Radical candor*' Kim Scott (2017) identifies four management style categories: obnoxious aggression, ruinous empathy, manipulative insincerity and radical candour (see *Table 3.5*) and considers how these styles impact on team building and team cohesion. In short, radical candour (the goal) as applied to student supervision and assessment requires the supervisor/assessor to set the right tone by offering direct and honest (constructive) criticism, being genuine when offering praise and being kind and respectful when delivering and receiving criticism (feedback), while remaining open to change. When applied to coaching conversations, candid feedback is more likely to have the intended impact on students in terms of their personal development than vague or superficial feedback or outright destructive criticism (Cantillon and Sargeant, 2008; Glover, 2000).

Table 3.5: Management styles (adapted from Scott, 2017)

Obnoxious aggression	**Ruinous empathy**
Known as brutal honesty (front stabbing) and includes direct challenges while failing to show you care about them personally, insincere praise and unkind criticism	Wanting to spare someone's feelings so failing to tell them something they need to know; you care personally but fail to challenge directly; includes non-specific praise so the person is unclear about what went well, vague or sugar-coated criticism or saying nothing at all: 'if nothing good to say, say nothing at all'
Manipulative insincerity	**Radical candour**
Known as 'backstabbing' and includes insincere praise, being complimentary face-to-face but criticising behind the person's back; you neither care personally nor challenge directly and can be passive aggressive	You care personally and challenge directly while being sincere, kind, specific and clear

 ACTIVITY 3.7

Structured feedback models can be useful tools to use when starting a feedback conversation with your student. What feedback models have you used or are you aware of?

There is an outline answer at the end of the chapter. More examples are also offered in *Chapter 5*.

3.5 COACHING SPECTRUM

 TOP TIP

It is useful at this point to introduce the coaching spectrum, a tool that can be applied by supervisors and assessors to truly listen to what the student is saying and to engage with meaningful coaching conversations and giving feedback. Applying the coaching spectrum allows you to draw together and practice all of the coaching skills introduced to you so far.

Coaching approaches range from directive to non-directive, as can be seen in the coaching spectrum (*Figure 3.2*).

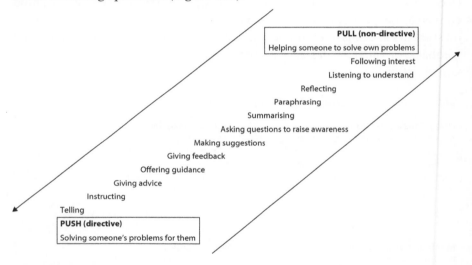

Figure 3.2: Coaching spectrum (adapted from Downey, 2014).

Traditionally the push or directive approaches are those employed by mentors, and non-directive or pull styles are those used by coaches. Both ends of the scale are equally important and practice supervisors should remain flexible in the style used. This will be determined through coaching conversations where the level of knowledge and skills of the student are established. This in turn will help to clarify the level of support that students require at any given time throughout their placement or indeed their programme. That is to say, a student who is new to placement and has never experienced a particular field of practice or performed a specific skill before will likely require a more directive approach where they are given instruction, advice or told how to do something. For more experienced students, non-directive styles can be used where questioning and listening techniques as discussed earlier in this section can be implemented.

> ### ☑ ACTIVITY 3.8
>
> Reflect on your last supervision interaction with a student. Where were you on the spectrum of coaching? Facing the same situation again, what other part of the spectrum might you use and why?
> This is a personal reflective activity, so no answer guide is provided.

Next, we explore the qualities of the supervisor who effectively applies coaching conversations.

3.6 EXPLORING THE QUALITIES OF THE SUPERVISOR WHO EFFECTIVELY APPLIES COACHING CONVERSATIONS

Holding coaching conversations is a skill that can be taught, and people can be educated to effectively engage with coaching conversations. However, there are qualities that people possess that allow them to deepen the effectiveness of the coaching conversations that they offer. These qualities are intrinsic and not so easy to instil as the knowledge and skill, but can develop over time and can be dependent on the experiences of individuals.

> ### ☑ ACTIVITY 3.9
>
> Refer to *Activity 3.2* and your definition of coaching. Reflect on your definition together with what you have learned about effective questioning, listening and providing feedback. Apply your knowledge by listing the qualities that you feel that an effective practice supervisor or assessor should demonstrate when using coaching conversations.
> This is a personal reflective activity, so no answer guide is provided.

3.6.1 Coaching qualities

Provided below are coaching qualities that when applied by the practice supervisor and assessor can help unlock student's potential for learning and achieving NMC programme outcomes and proficiencies:

A desire to help others and ability to motivate It goes without saying that to get the best out of a student you must be willing to invest in that person and demonstrate the skills to motivate them in their progress. To be effective in holding coaching conversations there is a need to recognise the achievement of others and to celebrate this to further encourage them.

Coachable To be coachable yourself indicates an openness to self-development, and an understanding of the processes and traits that act as a role model to others.

Respected/lead by example It is essential that as a supervisor or assessor you lead by example. Would you use a fitness coach who was unfit themselves? As an effective person who holds coaching conversations, you need to excel in your field of expertise and utilise this to your advantage and to motivate others; for example, making clear to students how you work within *The Code* (NMC, 2018c), promoting person-centred care.

Non-judgemental Being non-judgemental is one of the fundamental skills of being a nurse and indeed is a transferable quality to that of somebody who can use coaching conversations. As a supervisor or assessor, you are allowing students to express their thoughts, ideas and feelings openly and encouraging them to make decisions/actions for themselves. To be judgemental may result in a 'closed' student who is unwilling to engage in deeper exploration of concepts. It is a fact of life that you will hold your own opinions but for coaching conversations to be successful these must be put aside and the interests of your student must be the priority.

Honesty To develop good relationships honestly is invaluable. However, radical candour as previously explored in this chapter should be considered when giving feedback. Feedback should be specific and sincere while being kind. It is important that feedback is clear but still does not demotivate the recipient or cross boundaries by becoming personal.

✎ ACTIVITY 3.10

Building from *Activity 3.9*, reflect on the following key areas:
1. What qualities do you think you have that will help you to hold effective coaching conversations?
2. Are these innate qualities or have you developed them over time?
3. Could you develop any other qualities required?

This is a personal reflective activity, so no answer guide is provided.

3.7 CLINICAL LEADERSHIP DEVELOPMENT THROUGH ENGAGING IN COACHING CONVERSATIONS

One of the many benefits of adopting a coaching approach to supervision and assessment is promoting clinical leadership development.

Clinical leadership can be defined as: "providing excellent patient and client care through undertaking service improvement" (Chadwick and

Leigh, 2018, p. 120) and is a key component part of the role of every nurse or midwife who contributes to excellent patient and/or client care.

Developing students' clinical leadership relies on appropriate support offered from within the clinical environment and that students as learners are allowed to practise autonomously but in a safe and supported manner. West *et al.* (2015) concluded that preparation of healthcare staff in effective leadership skills is fundamental to improvements in health outcomes. The WHO (2020) also sees the value of nursing leadership when it is used to influence health policy formulation and decision-making.

Supervisors and assessors using coaching conversations can promote clinical leadership development through providing a conducive environment for students to gain independence and demonstrate leadership abilities when working within the multidisciplinary team and, as they progress through their programme of study, leading the team. This approach to leadership development supports students to become more confident in their own decision-making abilities.

When developing the student's clinical leadership, the supervisor as coach must ensure that patient safety is paramount. Use of a situational leadership model such as Hersey and Blanchard (1982) can assist the coach in knowing what level of support or delegation is suitable for each learner. Situational leadership can be used as a tool by the coach to apply the core concepts of coaching such as questioning, active listening and providing feedback to adapt the amount of autonomy given to the student that is dependent upon their current level of skills and knowledge alongside their willingness and motivation (see *Table 3.6*).

Table 3.6: Application of the Hersey and Blanchard (1982) situational leadership model

Student level of competence and motivation	Leadership style suggested
Learner has little ability or experience and lacks willingness or confidence	**Directive/Telling** Coach gives instruction and guidance to student and closely observes progress
Learner lacks ability but is keen to learn and practise	**Coaching/Selling** Coach explains procedures and rationales and is available to offer support to the learner
Learner is able and experienced but may lack motivation or confidence	**Supporting/Participating** Coach encourages learner to be involved by increasing confidence or enthusiasm
Learner is capable, confident and keen	**Delegating** Coach gives responsibility to the learner who will plan own goals and practise independently

Use of the effective questioning techniques discussed earlier will give the clinical coach the confidence in understanding the student learner's level of knowledge, ability and motivation. Coaching approaches may encourage supervisors to give students more independence when delivering and managing care, which in turn will allow the learner to feel more competent and ready to transition to a qualified professional more smoothly.

Thomson *et al.* (2017) discussed that some final placement students can feel ill-prepared for registration, which can be due to the lack of opportunity to develop their leadership and management skills. When supervisors use coaching conversations, students are engaged in their own learning and are given a suitable level of responsibility with their own patient allocation while reassured that there is an experienced supervisor monitoring their care. This enables the student to practise independently while feeling secure in the knowledge that there is a registrant available for them to discuss any concerns. The level of responsibility and leadership can be increased during the placement so that they feel included as a valuable team member, offering support to other learners and clearly demonstrating that they are achieving their NMC programme learning outcomes and proficiencies.

The next part of this chapter situates the core concepts of coaching conversations within a clinical coaching model. Using the GM Synergy model as an example, you will next apply a coaching model in clinical practice that sets out coach–student expectations and facilitates student learning, clinical leadership development and promotes wellbeing. The example provided is for nursing students but the model can be adapted to all undergraduate programmes that lead to NMC registration.

3.8 THE GM SYNERGY COACHING MODEL

Four Greater Manchester universities (see *Box 3.1*) provide undergraduate nursing programmes situated within Greater Manchester. Equipping Greater Manchester nursing students with exemplary clinical leadership skills is reliant on the practical component of their educational programme taking place in a supportive clinical environment. Aspiring nurse leaders should be supported to flourish in order that the future nursing workforce has the right leadership knowledge, skills and behaviours required to make sound clinical and non-clinical decisions that will empower nurses and strengthen nursing in decades to come. This in turn provides the optimum condition for delivering exemplary patient care.

Box 3.1: Four Greater Manchester universities

| University of Salford (UoS) |
| University of Manchester (UoM) |
| University of Bolton (UoB) |
| Manchester Metropolitan University (MMU) |

The Greater Manchester universities have a strong relationship and history of collaboration. Since 2009, Greater Manchester hospital Trusts, the four universities and Health Education England (HEE) have worked together as the Greater Manchester Practice Education Group – the aim is to operationalise the practice component of the undergraduate nursing programme. The strength of this group lies in the expertise and passion of its members who are all committed to providing the best opportunities for student learning when engaging in clinical practice.

Influenced by evidence from the Willis Commission (Willis, 2015) on the future of nursing education that provided evidence of the Collaborative Learning in Practice model (CLiP) and our own practice, the team also identified coaching as an effective model for student nurse support in practice. In 2016/17 members from the Greater Manchester Practice Education Group attended a study day facilitated by the University of East Anglia who had developed the coaching model (CLiP) and visited the Lancashire Teaching Trust who had implemented the model.

The vision was clear from the outset that any new model would continue to standardise Greater Manchester resources while at the same time promote flexibility and freedom in the diverse clinical contexts and healthcare organisations. In this way, it was recognised that there was a need to create a bespoke model that would be responsive to the differing context and needs of each hospital Trust and university involved, thus complementing the Greater Manchester transformation agenda.

The GM Synergy coaching model is summarised in *Figure 3.3.*

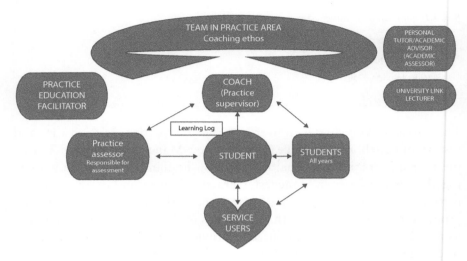

Figure 3.3: The GM Synergy coaching model.

3.8.1 Setting up the GM Synergy coaching model

The four universities and healthcare organisations worked in partnership to identify GM Synergy placement areas and agreed coach–student expectations and what effective supervision and assessment would look like. Under the supervision of a practice supervisor who uses a coaching approach, the student would be expected to become actively involved in all aspects of nursing care. Students, taking into account previous learning experiences and learning needs, develop their ability to reflect on their advancing knowledge, skills and behaviours (Leigh *et al.*, 2019).

ACTIVITY 3.11

Place yourself in the situation where you are thinking about introducing a coaching model in one clinical placement area. What educational support would be required?

An answer guide has been developed by an experienced practice education facilitator who reflects on their experiences of providing support in preparation for opening a GM Synergy coaching placement in a large NHS Foundation Trust.

A typical GM Synergy day is described below.

3.8.2 GM Synergy: a typical day

GM Synergy placement areas are allocated undergraduate student nurses (often, but not always, a combination of first-, second- and third-year) though not all will be on duty at the same time. Placements are situated within hospitals (spanning adult and child and intermediate care settings) and attended by adult and children and young people fields of practice. Many practice areas are split into 'bays' and there may be one or more bays that will operate the GM Synergy model at the same time, allowing a large volume of students to be accommodated. This contrasts with non-Synergy areas where student allocation can be as low as one. This high volume of students is required to provide the peer teaching and learning opportunities. At the start of the shift, students meet with their coach for the day (who is predominantly the practice supervisor), the ideal ratio being four students to one coach (Leigh *et al.*, 2019), to discuss their learning needs for the day. Students complete their learning log, focusing on specific learning objectives related to their placement learning objectives. Students provide care to patients with direct support and supervision from the coach. The practice assessor will observe the student and conduct the summative assessments.

Peer teaching and learning also takes place between the first-, second- and third-year students. At set times throughout the shift the coach and students review learning based around the students' learning objectives, critically reflecting on what they have learnt and continuously planning for the next learning opportunity. Other key practice-based education roles that support effective GM Synergy delivery include the practice education facilitator and academic assessor. These roles have been explored in *Chapter 2*.

The GM Synergy Model is continuing to evolve, providing the multi-professional coaching experiences for all learners that take place from within the range of health and social care settings. Key to the emergent model is the learning with and from each other.

Provided next are *Top Tips* when planning supervision and assessment for student nurses who for the shift are engaging with the GM Synergy model.

TOP TIP

Supervision and assessment with the coach at the start of the shift:
- Coach meets with the students to discuss the plan for the day and patient allocation; this is dependent on the students' prior knowledge, experience and learning needs as discussed with the practice supervisor
- Negotiate frequency of reviews/how often you will catch up
- Explore learning opportunities – following the patient journey
- Consider any proficiencies and professional values to be assessed by the practice assessor
- Consider if the academic assessor is to be involved (this role is discussed in detail in *Chapter 2*)

TOP TIP

Supervision and assessment with the coach at the mid-point of the shift:
- Coach and student review progress and implement changes if required
- Practice supervisor and other personnel will be available to support the coach and teach/guide as required
- Feedback from coach, discuss evidence gathered and skills being developed, adapt or build on original plan if necessary
- Confirm actions for the remainder of the shift
- Practice supervisor, student and practice assessor discuss summative assessment (if appropriate)

TOP TIP

Student supervision and assessment with the coach at the end of the shift:

Coach:
- Reviews the day with student and provides feedback
- Completes the learning log and reflects on the day, discussing outcomes with practice supervisor and/or practice assessor

Student:
- Evaluates own progress and provides feedback to the coach
- Reflects on the day with practice supervisor/practice assessor and plans for the next learning opportunity
- Practice supervisor, student and practice assessor discuss summative assessment (if appropriate)

3.9 SUMMARY

This chapter has defined coaching and has provided you with the opportunity to understand the differences between coaching and mentoring. Through engaging in a series of activities, you have examined the core concepts of coaching conversations that, when applied to supervision and assessment of students, effectively facilitate student learning. The qualities of the effective coach in clinical practice have been explored. Using the GM Synergy model as a case study example, you have knowledge of a coaching model in clinical practice that clearly applies the supervisor and assessor roles set out in the NMC (2018b) *Part 2: Standards for student supervision and assessment.* The model, however, is transferable to all undergraduate NMC programmes that lead to registration. Through clearly identifying the coach–student expectations, there is the opportunity to promote students' clinical leadership development, achievement of NMC programme proficiencies and student wellbeing.

RECOMMENDED FURTHER READING

Dinkins, C.S. and Cangelosi, P.R. (2019) Putting Socrates back in Socratic method: Theory-based debriefing in the nursing classroom. *Nursing Philosophy*, **20**(2): e12240. doi: 10.1111/nup.12240

Access the following link to find out more about the NHS Leadership Academy Healthcare Leadership Model: www.leadershipacademy.nhs. uk/resources/healthcare-leadership-model/

REFERENCES

Andrews, M. and Roberts, D. (2003) Supporting student nurses learning in and through clinical practice: the role of the clinical guide. *Nurse Education Today*, **23**: 471–81.

Cambridge dictionary. Cambridge University Press. Available at: https:// dictionary.cambridge.org/ (accessed 14 August 2020).

Cantillon, P. and Sargeant, J. (2008) Giving feedback in clinical settings. *BMJ*, **337**: a1961. doi: 10.1136/bmj.a1961

Center for Creative Leadership (2019) *Immediately improve your talent development.* Available at: www.ccl.org/articles/leading-effectively-articles/hr-pipeline-a-quick-win-to-improve-your-talent-development-process/ (accessed 14 August 2020).

Chadwick, A. and Leigh J. (2018) Identifying and developing clinical leadership in relation to transition. In: Darvill, A., Stephenson, M.

and Leigh, J.A. (editors) *Transition to nursing practice: from student to registered nurse.* Sage.

Clynes, M.P. and Raftery, S.E.C. (2008) Feedback: An essential element of student learning in clinical practice. *Nurse Education in Practice,* 8: 404–11.

Downey, M. (2014) *Effective modern coaching: the principles and art of successful business coaching.* LID.

Duffy, K. (2013) Deciding to fail: Nurse mentors' experiences of managing a failed practice assessment. *Journal of Practice Teaching and Learning* 11(3): 36–58. doi: 10.1921/2102110304

Glover, P.A. (2000) Feedback. I listened, reflected and utilised: third year nursing students' perceptions and use of feedback in the clinical setting. *International Journal of Nursing Practice,* 6: 247–52.

Hersey, P. and Blanchard, K. (1982) *Management of organizational behavior – utilizing human resources.* 4th edition. Prentice Hall.

Kimsey-House, H., Kimsey-House, K., Sandahl, P. and Whitworth, L. (2011) *Co-active coaching: Changing business, transforming lives.* 3rd edition. Nicholas Brealey.

Kline, N. (2015) *More time to think: the power of independent thinking.* Octopus.

Leigh, J.A., Littlewood, L. and Lyons, G. (2019) Reflection on creating a coaching approach to student nurse clinical leadership development. *British Journal of Nursing,* 28(17): 1124–28. doi: 10.12968/ bjon.2019.28.17.1124

McCarthy, B., Trace, A., O'Donovan, M. *et al.* (2018) Nursing and midwifery students' stress and coping during their undergraduate education programmes: an integrative review. *Nurse Education Today,* 61: 197–209.

Nursing and Midwifery Council (2018a) *Future nurse: Standards of proficiency for registered nurses.* NMC. Available at: www.nmc.org. uk/globalassets/sitedocuments/education-standards/future-nurse-proficiencies.pdf (accessed 13 August 2020).

Nursing and Midwifery Council (2018b) *Realising professionalism: Part 2: Standards for student supervision and assessment.* NMC. Available at: www.nmc.org.uk/globalassets/sitedocuments/ education-standards/student-supervision-assessment.pdf (accessed 13 August 2020).

Nursing and Midwifery Council (2018c) *The Code: Professional standards of practice and behaviour for nurses, midwives and nursing associates.* NMC. Available at: www.nmc.org.uk/globalassets/sitedocuments/nmc-publications/nmc-code.pdf (accessed 29 September 2020).

Pendleton, D., Schofield, T., Tate, P. and Havelock, P. (2003) *The new consultation: developing doctor–patient communication.* Oxford University Press.

Royal College of Nursing (2017) *Guidance for mentors of nursing and midwifery students.* RCN. Available at: https://bhcic.co.uk/wp-content/uploads/2018/07/RCN-Guidance-for-Mentors-of-Nurseing-and-Midwifery-Students-.pdf (accessed 28 September 2020).

Scott, K. (2017) *Radical candor: how to be a great boss without losing your humanity.* Pan Macmillan.

Starr, J. (2016) *The coaching manual: the definitive guide to the process, principles and skills of personal coaching.* 4th edition. Pearson.

Straker, D. (2010) *Changing minds in detail.* 2nd edition. Syque.

Thomson, R., Docherty, A. and Duffy, R. (2017) Nursing students' experiences of mentorship in their final placement. *British Journal of Nursing,* **26(9):** 514–21.

Watson, R., Rehman, S. and Ali, P.A. (2017) Stressors affecting nursing students in Pakistan. *International Nursing Review,* **64:** 536–43.

West, M., Armit, K., Loewenthal, L. *et al.* (2015) Leadership and leadership development in health care: The evidence base. The King's Fund. Available at: https://www.kingsfund.org.uk/publications/leadership-and-leadership-development-health-care (accessed 18 August 2020).

Whitmore, J. (2017) *Coaching for performance: The principles and practice of coaching and leadership.* 5th edition. Nicholas Brealey.

Willis G.P. (2015) *Shape of caring: A review of the future education and training of registered nurses and care assistants.* Health Education England. Available at: www.hee.nhs.uk/sites/default/files/documents/2348-Shape-of-caring-review-FINAL.pdf (accessed 13 August 2020).

World Health Organization (2020) *State of the world's nursing 2020.* London: WHO. Available at: www.who.int/publications/i/item/9789240003279 (accessed 30 November 2020).

ACTIVITY ANSWER GUIDES

ACTIVITY 3.2

Provided in the table are benefits and risks that you may have identified:

Benefits of adopting a coaching approach	Risks of adopting a coaching approach
Students: improved performance, motivation, commitment, personal growth, quality of life, work–life balance, sense of purpose, satisfaction, communication, relationships **Practice supervisor as coach:** improved self-awareness, listening, satisfaction (due to making a difference), intellectual challenge, skills (e.g. questioning), issue awareness, management of people and teams	**Students:** may not feel ready for their increased responsibility **Practice supervisor as coach:** may not feel adequately prepared and supported in their role

Strategies to address the associated risks include ensuring that the student and practice supervisor as coach are all fully prepared for their roles and that effective communication takes place between the coach, supervisor and assessor.

ACTIVITY 3.6

Techniques to demonstrate you have both listened and heard what has been said:

Paraphrasing	Using your own words to express what was said (or written) by another person
Summarising	Giving a brief overview of whole conversation/discussion
Reflecting back	Repeating words back in exactly the same way as the other person said them; can be done not just by reflecting back the word(s) and how they were spoken but also the body language used by the person speaking Reflecting back is like holding up a mirror to that person, so if they fold their arms when using a particular word or phrase you would do the same This raises awareness in the speaker as they may not be aware of their body language or the tone they use with certain words
Mirroring	When done with intent, rather like reflecting back body language, it can demonstrate you are listening – not just the words spoken but to the non-verbal language Unintentional mirroring often occurs when someone (the listener) is engrossed in what is being said and subconsciously they begin to mirror the body language of the person speaking
Leaning in	Research shows that leaning forward when listening tends to increase the verbal output of the person speaking

ACTIVITY 3.7

There are a number of feedback models that can be used; two which are commonly used in practice are summarised here.

Pendleton's rules

	What went well	Improvement areas	Action plan	Summary
Coachee	Explains what went well	Explains what could be done better	Explains action plan	Summarises key points
Coach	Comments on what went well	Comments on what could be done better	Approves action plan with modifications if required	Comments as appropriate

Pendleton et al. *(2003)*

Situation, behaviour, impact model

Situation	Be clear and define the when and where of the situation to which you are referring; this provides context to the person you are giving feedback to
Behaviour	Describe specific behaviours (actions) you want to address; comment only on what you directly observed, stating facts and avoiding assumptions
Impact	Use 'I' statements to describe what impact these behaviours/actions had on you and/or others
Once feedback is delivered, encourage the person to reflect on the situation in order to understand and learn.	

Center for Creative Leadership (2019)

ACTIVITY 3.11

A clinically based lead person was identified to work with the pilot areas assisting them with training staff around the GM Synergy coaching model – providing information, advice, guidance and resources on an ongoing basis to assist the placements to establish and implement the model during its initial introduction.

During the initial introduction of the model to the placement area, sufficient learners were allocated to each placement after being prepared by the four universities. The GM Synergy lead visited the placement areas to support inductions and then regularly to support staff and learners with queries and reinforce the use of coaching by identifying coaching opportunities, offering advice around allocation of learners to placement tasks and responsibilities to support their learning and peer support, and ensure effective supervision of learners involved in a hands-on approach to learning was maintained. The Synergy lead worked with placement staff to organise off duties ensuring learner skill mix allocated to off duty were being coordinated effectively to enhance the opportunities for peer support and leadership development.

CHAPTER 4

INTERPROFESSIONAL SUPERVISION OF STUDENT LEARNING

Joanna Barlow, Leigh Campbell, Zoe Tilley and Jo Pierce

4.1 INTRODUCTION

The new Nursing and Midwifery Council (NMC) standards for student supervision and assessment (NMC, 2018c) state that nursing and midwifery students can be supervised by any registered health and social care professional working within a healthcare environment. These professionals may be registered with regulatory bodies such as the NMC, Health and Care Professions Council (HCPC) or General Medical Council (GMC).

This may initially suggest an expectation that all healthcare professionals will be required to supervise nursing and midwifery students for considerable blocks of learning within the practice environment. However, further exploration of the standards suggests this is not the case. It is proposed that learning experiences should have: "an interdisciplinary and interprofessional learning context, including learning with and from other professions where appropriate" (NMC, 2019).

This chapter will explore the role that other healthcare professionals can play in supervising and educating nursing and midwifery students, and how this may be implemented in practice. To help you make the most of this chapter, you should be familiar with the NMC standards as these will be used throughout to reference, underpin and illustrate key discussion points. In line with this, the terms used within these standards (such as practice supervisor) will be referred to within this chapter for clarity and consistency, though it is recognised that different health and social care professionals use different terminology (Emerson, 2004).

After reading this chapter you will be able to:
- Identify a range of health and social care professionals that work with student nurses and midwives and who contribute to the delivery of safe and effective patient care

- Begin to have interprofessional team discussions about what each person can add to the student's learning journey
- Identify specific knowledge and skills that interprofessional colleagues have that students can learn from
- Have an increased awareness of the role of interprofessional clinical supervisors.

4.2 INTERPROFESSIONAL LEARNING IN THE HEALTHCARE ENVIRONMENT

ACTIVITY 4.1

Reflect on a situation when you have supervised a student from within your own profession. Did you ever arrange for them to shadow other professions in the healthcare environment? If so, why did you do this? What did you expect the student to gain from this experience?

This is a personal reflective activity, so no answer guide is provided.

Arranging time for students to observe and work alongside other professions within your practice area provides insight into the role and responsibilities of other healthcare professionals. Additionally, the student can experience how the interdisciplinary team (IDT) works together to deliver the best quality care for the patient.

The concept of interprofessional learning (IPL) and interprofessional education (IPE), and their use in clinical practice, is not new. Established in 1987, the Centre for the Advancement of Interprofessional Education (CAIPE), a UK-based charity, defines IPE as: "occasions when two or more professions learn with, from and about each other to improve collaboration and the quality of care" (Centre for the Advancement of Interprofessional Education, 2019; Reeves *et al.*, 2013).

ACTIVITY 4.2

Think about the team that you currently work in. How many different professions do you regularly interact with to enable you to deliver care to your patients? What have you learnt from and about these other professions? How does this contribute to the care and management of patients?

This is a personal reflective activity, so no answer guide is provided.

In November 2001, the Department of Health (DH) developed a framework to support the vision of lifelong learning, supporting staff to acquire new skills and realise their potential (DH, 2001). The primary aim of the framework was to ensure patients and their families were cared for by a qualified and motivated workforce. At the time there was great emphasis put on the need for shared learning and effective team working between professions and staff groups. Understanding the role of other healthcare professions was considered imperative for delivering quality care to patients. Furthermore, it was stated that this should be included from the earliest point possible in healthcare education, in both academic and practice settings. The framework was further updated in 2007, but the essence of the message remains (DH/CAIPE, 2007). Furthermore, the *NHS long term plan* (Department of Health and Social Care, 2019) recognises interdisciplinary education as a means to producing the flexible workforce, something required if the key ambitions for the National Health Service (NHS) over the next 10 years are to be met.

Recommendations for promoting shared learning and greater understanding of other professions' roles have been made as a result of high-profile cases. Examples include inquiries into children's heart surgery at Bristol Royal Infirmary (DH, 2002) and poor standards of patient care and serious failings within Mid-Staffordshire NHS Trust (Francis, 2013). The Interprofessional Education Collaborative Expert Panel (2011) stated that the fast-changing healthcare system calls for innovations in health professional education to enhance interprofessional (IP) practice skills to improve care and population health outcomes and reduce costs. Professional bodies have incorporated these recommendations into their standards for education and training to ensure students on healthcare courses are given opportunities to learn from, and with, other professions.

ACTIVITY 4.3

In your experience as a healthcare professional, can you think of a team you have worked in with an effective interdisciplinary approach to patient care? Why did it work well? Have you experience of a team where interdisciplinary working was lacking and why this might have been the case?

This is a personal reflective activity, so no answer guide is provided.

It could be argued that the need for interdisciplinary teamwork is further increasing due to people living longer with multiple long-term conditions and complex needs; no single profession will be able to optimally meet these challenging needs working in isolation. Part of the solution is to understand, embrace and implement IDT working, with the aim of promoting a collaborative, positive, safe and caring environment.

Some of the positive characteristics of an effective IDT you may have considered in the above exercise may have included: a clear leader who listens, good communication skills, motivation to work together, a culture of trust, or a clear set of values and beliefs. These are among the factors recognised as valuable characteristics of an IDT (Nancarrow *et al.*, 2013) and provide a good framework for teams to work within.

We have considered why collaborating and communicating with other professions can benefit patient safety and care. Let us now consider how this can be implemented into clinical practice, through educating and working alongside healthcare learners.

4.3 INTERPROFESSIONAL SUPERVISION IN HEALTHCARE TO FOSTER LEARNING

Studies within healthcare education have shown IPL to be a positive experience in both classroom and practice settings. It has been reported that learning topics, which can be directly applied to clinical practice, are considered most effective, allowing each profession to learn the value and significance of each other's contribution to patient care, with an emphasis on interactive and active learning (Morison *et al.*, 2003). This is further supported by Reeves *et al.* (2016) who suggested that for IPL to be effective, it needs to be context specific, i.e. carried out within an environment that best represents learners' current or future practice. This should involve the agreement of clear goals achieved through the most effective teaching method, and should allow professions to recognise and value the similarities and differences between healthcare roles (McPherson *et al.*, 2001).

Occupational therapy (OT) has long embraced alternative approaches to supervising learners in healthcare. Role-emerging placements enable the OT learner to spend time in a setting where there is currently no OT provision. Learners are tasked with identifying a role for OT within that environment and can be supervised on a daily basis by a different profession, but may also have off-site supervision (or long-arm supervision) from an OT (Overton *et al.*, 2009). For this model to be successful, it is suggested that training is provided for placement supervisors to ensure clear goals and outcomes are identified.

The introduction of the NMC standards of student supervision (NMC, 2018c) provides an opportunity to rethink how IPL can happen in practice for nursing students. As previously discussed, it may already be common practice to provide insight visits for students to work alongside, or shadow, other professionals. There is now an opportunity to formalise this process, allowing nursing and midwifery students to achieve their learning outcomes, which could also benefit all other healthcare learners.

4.4 ROLE OF THE ALLIED HEALTH PROFESSIONAL AS A PRACTICE SUPERVISOR

To enable the supervision of students within their own profession, allied health professionals (AHPs) are required to complete a practice supervisor education programme. Specific skills and knowledge taught on the programme will also inform student nursing or midwifery practice, with likely topic areas covered including: an understanding of how people learn, managing the learning environment, facilitating learning, and acting as a role model, which will contribute to the promotion of IPL (Emerson, 2004). It is important to remember that AHPs are expected to contribute to student learning only within their scope of practice (NMC, 2018c). The role as an AHP or other healthcare professional, such as doctor, when taking on the role of practice supervisor for a nursing or midwifery student will be able to:

- Provide a safe, trusting learning environment where students are facilitated and feel empowered to achieve their learning outcomes
- Serve as a role model for safe and effective practice
- Provide the student with an insight into the role of their profession
- Highlight opportunities for shared learning.

The following sections will explore how AHPs and other healthcare professionals can incorporate these areas into their own clinical context and practice.

4.4.1 Creating an effective learning environment

 SCENARIO 4.1

Jenny is a student nurse. She is to spend the day with the OT team to learn about their role with patients on a busy orthopaedic ward. When Jenny arrives at the specified time of 0830 hours, the OT is not on the ward. Jenny does not recognise any of the staff on the ward. She is not sure where she should stand or if she should go and look for the OT. No one has looked in her direction or asked if they can help her.

> ### ✍ ACTIVITY 4.4
>
> How would you feel if you were Jenny? Have you experienced anything like this, as either a student or a professional?
> This is a personal reflective activity, so no answer guide is provided.

Attitudes and behaviours within a workplace can greatly influence learning. A sense of belonging is vital to ensure students feel valued and accepted within a team. Being made to feel welcome, included in patient care and social inclusion were found to increase confidence and lead to an improved placement experience (Levett-Jones *et al.*, 2009b). Indeed, Jack *et al.* (2018) suggest the importance of understanding the student nurse perspective and explore ways in which their feelings of belongingness might be enhanced in the clinical area. In *Scenario 4.1*, Jenny could have been made to feel more welcome if any one of the staff had acknowledged her presence, by asking who she was waiting for or offering her a quiet place to sit while she waited for the OT to arrive (*Scenario 4.2*).

In a positive learning environment, students will feel psychologically safe: confident in speaking out, engaged in the learning context and free to interact without fear of judgement (Bynum and Haque, 2016; Oandasan and Reeves, 2005). An environment instilling feeling of hostility towards learners may encourage the wrong behaviours. Fisher and Kiernan (2019) state that students have a strong desire to 'fit in' to the clinical environment to 'survive' the placement. As a result of this, if the student feels 'unsafe', they may not feel able to raise concerns around their own learning requirements, or more importantly standards of care. Standard 3.2 of the NMC standards framework for education states that students should be empowered and supported to become "resilient, caring, reflective lifelong learners" and acquire the skills to work in an IP team (NMC, 2018b). The learning environment is discussed earlier in this book and is further explored in *Chapter 9*.

> ### 📂 SCENARIO 4.2
>
> The OT has arrived on the ward and immediately finds Jenny and introduces herself. They go and find a quiet space on the ward to discuss the plan for the day.

ACTIVITY 4.5

Taking on an AHP or other health professional role (apart from nursing and midwifery), what conversations might you have with Jenny to ensure a positive learning experience? What will you need to ask her? What questions might Jenny have for you?

An answer guide is provided at the end of the chapter.

4.4.2 Facilitating the achievement of learning outcomes

The student should be at the centre of the learning experience. They should be empowered to take responsibility for their learning, while maintaining a safe environment and ensuring quality of patient care and management.

There are several ways learning outcomes (LOs) might be best achieved; it is a shared decision between the practice supervisor and student about the approach taken. These may involve direct patient care, discussions, reflections, peer-to-peer learning, classroom-based learning or simulation, and may be selected depending on your role and the knowledge or skills to be learnt.

 SCENARIO 4.3

Continuing with the scenario of Jenny, she has identified the following LO she would like to achieve during her current clinical placement:

Take appropriate action to reduce or minimise pain or discomfort (NMC, 2018a, Annexe B: 3.5)

 ACTIVITY 4.6

Who might be the best educator or practice supervisor to assist Jenny in achieving this outcome and what teaching approaches may be utilised?

An answer guide is provided at the end of the chapter.

You could also consider the possibility of students learning together or from each other. Hood *et al.* (2014) reported that students from many professions, working together in a ward environment, learned the practice of IDT collaboration in a more effective manner. Independently managing the care of a patient gave them a sense of belonging and provided insight into their future healthcare professional role.

Creating an optimal learning environment is essential for anyone, at any point in their career, to ensure good communication and safe management of patients. Establishing this for students is imperative to ensure learning can take place.

To understand more about how you can help develop a sense of belonging for your learners and create a positive learning environment, you may want to read the following from the reference list: Jack *et al.* (2018) and Levett-Jones and Lathlean (2009a). The latter reference, for example, describes the importance of creating a sense of belonging for students, and that unless and until students feel like they belong to the team, their learning can be hampered.

4.4.3 Role models and advocacy in the context of practice education

To be an effective role model in practice education and advocate for IPL, it is useful to explore the key concepts and ideologies in play. Johnson states that:

> "A role model is a person looked to by others as an example to be imitated. They possess qualities that we would like to have, and we try to emulate them. They make us want to be better at what we do. They inspire us, motivate us, and encourage us to try a little harder to be a better nurse or educator". (Johnson, 2015)

Within this definition, the following eight characteristics of effective role models were identified:
1. Passion
2. Integrity
3. Excellence
4. Positive choice making
5. Confidence
6. Optimism
7. Resilience / ability to overcome obstacles
8. Generosity.

(Johnson, 2015)

Johnson explains some of the nuances of each characteristic within the context of being a role model within healthcare; you may want to read more about this (see *References* for details).

ACTIVITY 4.7

Cast your mind back to when you were a student in clinical practice. Think of your supervisors. What attributes made them 'good' or 'bad' role models? Did they demonstrate any of the above characteristics? Reflect for a moment on how these influenced your learning.

Have you had an opportunity to supervise a student? If yes, reflect on which of the above characteristics you might have conveyed.

This is a personal reflective activity, so no answer guide is provided.

The standards of proficiency for nursing associates (NMC, 2018d) identifies the importance of being able to supervise and act as a role model to nursing associate students, healthcare support workers and those new to care roles, promoting reflection and providing constructive feedback. Davis (2013) suggests that working with role models and observing them in their roles is the start of 'professional socialisation'. According to Belinsky and Tataronis (2007), exposure to positive role models "facilitates the development of practices and beliefs that help to ensure the provision of high-quality care". It is also a means to embed within the student qualities such as behaviour, attitudes and values (Flynn, 2011).

To date, the literature around role modelling within healthcare tends to focus on uniprofessional role modelling. However, nursing and midwifery students can observe many members of the IDT during their education and the various influences they are exposed to can be good or bad, confusing, varied and complex (Hinton, 2014). Donaldson and Carter (2005) explored the value of role modelling in adult nursing practice education and found that all students experienced 'good' and 'bad' clinical role models. They identified role modelling as extremely important within the clinical learning environment. Students also agreed that it was not always the practice supervisor who provided good role modelling, but members of the wider IDT.

The importance of IP role modelling is investigated in a research report produced by the Health and Care Professions Council (HCPC) on *Professionalism in healthcare professionals* (HCPC, 2011). Role models were not limited to the student's own profession, but extended to other professions. The quotes below capture this:

> "*I think looking at other professions, not just podiatrists, but GPs, nurses, doctors, physios, dentists, how do they conduct themselves in a professional manner, what's their understanding of professionalism? Looking at how other people present themselves professionally, not just medically, but in business as well and just throughout general life*". (Podiatry student)

> *"Taking bits from all the different people that you meet...*
> *you'll see something and think that's really good, and then it's*
> *taking the best bits from everyone, saying they're really good*
> *at talking to the client and getting their attention, and then...*
> *they're really good at putting equipment together and this is*
> *the best way to do that...and I've learned a lot from other*
> *people in the team as well and I think that's really important".*
> (OT student)

The above examples illustrate that role modelling can be an extremely effective means of teaching and learning. So how can this be achieved? Cruess *et al.* (2008) suggest several strategies to improve role modelling. Among these are:

- Be aware of being a role model
- Show a positive attitude for what you do
- Facilitate reflection on clinical experiences including role modelling
- Work to improve the institutional culture.

As an AHP or other healthcare professional when supervising a student, whether from the same profession or a different one, it is important to be aware of the message you wish to be conveyed. IP role modelling is an opportunity to increase awareness and understanding of the role. It is also an opportunity to teach transferable skills, such as communication, empathy or compassion. These are explored in the following practice example (*Scenario 4.4*).

 SCENARIO 4.4

David is a third-year adult nursing student on his fifth week of placement on an oncology ward. His supervisor has arranged for him to spend the day with one of the ward physiotherapists, Anila.

Anila welcomes David with a smile and tells him they have a busy day of pre-ops and post-ops. She appears happy to have him join her for the day and both are keen to make the most of this learning opportunity. She takes a few minutes to ask David what his experience has been on the ward thus far and what he most wants to get out of their day together.

They first go and see Reggie, who is scheduled for a bowel resection tomorrow. Anila educates Reggie on pain management, chest care and what to expect in terms of mobilisation. During this interaction, Reggie becomes tearful. He apologises, attempting to brush it off quickly and asks Anila to carry on. Anila sits down, takes Reggie's hand and reassures him. He expresses anxiety around pain and how this will be managed. Anila reassures him the

SCENARIO 4.4 *(cont'd)*

doctors and nursing staff will do their absolute best to ensure he is as comfortable as possible. Knowing that David has had experience with patient-controlled anaesthesia (PCA) pumps, Anila asks him if he is happy to explain to Reggie how they work.

 ACTIVITY 4.8

Consider the above practice example. How does Anila make David feel at ease? Are there any transferable skills David will be able to use as a nursing student? Do you feel Anila was a good role model for David? If so, why?
An answer guide is provided at the end of the chapter.

According to Brandt (2018), students require structured learning from clinical team role models. For this to be the case, consistent team role models need to exist in practice. The concepts of team role modelling and IPL advocacy are examined further in the practice example (*Scenario 4.5*).

 SCENARIO 4.5

Gill is an OT student on her tenth week of placement in a neurological rehabilitation unit. Neil, a man who sustained an acquired brain injury 4 months ago, is being hoisted for all transfers and is fully dependent on a wheelchair for mobility. He is able to tolerate sitting out for 30 minutes. Neil has a tracheostomy tube *in situ*, but it is being capped off for short periods. During this time, he is working with the speech and language therapist (SLT), Catherine, on producing vocal sounds.

Catherine is due to see Neil today, but would ideally like him to be in his wheelchair for the session. When she arrives on the ward, Neil is just finishing his washing and dressing with Gill and Andy, a student nurse. Gill has been leading the session to demonstrate how much Neil is able to do for himself, using appropriate equipment and prompts. Catherine asks whether they might be able to hoist him into his wheelchair for her session which Gill and Andy are happy to do.

With Neil's consent, both students are keen to join the SLT session. Before the session starts, Catherine asks each student to: (1) consider one component of the intervention to reflect upon afterwards, and (2) identify one or two strategies observed during the session used to help Neil with his communication. After the session, Catherine carried out a 10-minute debrief to answer any questions and to highlight the key learning points.

ACTIVITY 4.9

Consider your own practice. Do you work within a team that advocates IPL? If yes, in what ways is this message conveyed? Could this be developed further? This is a personal reflective activity, so no answer guide is provided.

4.4.4 Knowledge of professional roles: identifying similarities and differences

We have discussed earlier in the chapter that IP working and education are not new concepts (DH, 2001; Department of Health and Social Care, 2019; McPherson *et al.*, 2001; Morison *et al.*, 2003; Oandasan and Reeves, 2005), though challenges with putting these into practice remain (Atwal, 2018; Gilligan *et al.*, 2014; Palese *et al.*, 2019). One of the challenges can be recognising, let alone utilising, opportunities for shared learning between professions.

IPL provides opportunities for shared learning, but the success of this relies on a number of factors. A systematic review examining midwives' and nurses' collaborative experience found negative experiences of IPE might be influenced by unclear roles, among other factors (Jackson *et al.*, 2016); therefore it might be useful to identify some of the ways in which professions are similar and where they differ.

Shared values, knowledge and approaches, such as empathetic communication and person-centred care, are considered key skills that all healthcare professionals learn and continue to develop, regardless of profession. However, specific clinical skills or areas of knowledge, such as carrying out an X-ray procedure, auscultation, applying a particular splint or prescribing an optimal walking aid, can be considered skills more appropriately learned through education by the most appropriate profession.

Let us first consider similarities between professions and how those working as AHP or other healthcare professional practice supervisors can help students first identify and then go on to use learning opportunities to develop these shared skills and knowledge. A practical way to illustrate this could be to carry out *Activity 4.10* with a variety of professionals and students.

ACTIVITY 4.10

What key knowledge and skills are required in the job of AHP to enable the delivery of a quality service to patients? Now review each person's list and highlight the ones that are the same, i.e. shared by other professionals, and those that are different. This exercise will be returned to later in the chapter.
This is a personal reflective activity, so no answer guide is provided.

Although each group and person carrying out this exercise will of course generate a different list, it is anticipated that each list would include care standards reflective of the seven platforms listed in the NMC standards of proficiency (NMC, 2018a). These include: being an accountable professional, promoting health and preventing ill health, assessing needs and planning care, providing and evaluating care, leading and managing (nursing) care, and working in teams and coordinating care (see the first reference in *Activity 4.11* for further details; Annexe A of this resource focuses on communication and relationship management skills and details a list of interpersonal and team working communication skills shared across all professions.

ACTIVITY 4.11

Review *Future nurse: Standards of proficiency for registered nurses*: www.nmc.org.uk/standards/standards-for-nurses/standards-of-proficiency-for-registered-nurses/ Consider how these standards apply in a specific area of work as an AHP.
Review the standards of proficiency for another healthcare professional: www.hcpc-uk.org/standards/standards-of-proficiency and highlight similarities between these and the nursing standards of proficiency.
An answer guide is not provided for this activity.

Annexe A of the NMC *Future nurse: Standards of proficiency for registered nurses* explains how registered nurses must be able to demonstrate the ability to communicate and manage relationships with people of all ages with a range of mental, physical, cognitive and behavioural health challenges. Radiology offers an ideal learning opportunity for students to observe, reflect upon and practise ways in which patient care can be optimised. Radiographers will encompass patients with wide-ranging health challenges and must develop their own way of assessing and resolving communication barriers, often with minimal (if any) prior knowledge of the patients' specific communication difficulty. First, let us consider a commonly encountered chest X-ray examination and think about the potential for learning core skills required for all healthcare professionals.

An X-ray procedure could be considered routine; however, each is unique as the approach is patient-centred, requiring the radiographer to have an armoury of approaches available to them. Often in radiology, patients can be distressed, confused, agitated, aggressive and often in pain. The use of de-escalation strategies and techniques are required to ensure the examination can proceed safely. This is a good learning opportunity for students to observe and identify helpful strategies they can later develop in elements of required nursing practice as identified in Annexe A of the NMC standards: (be able to) "identify the need for and manage a range of alternative communication techniques" (NMC, 2018a, Annexe A, p. 29, Standard 2.5). Radiology may seem significantly different to other disciplines within the hospital. However, there are many common themes shared between professions and disciplines, such as the patient being at the centre of their care. Although taking an X-ray may appear task orientated, this must be achieved safely, with compassion, decency and dignity.

You will have discussed and considered shared knowledge, skills and areas of practice through the exercise and worked example above. These core skills, previously highlighted as being critical for delivering quality healthcare, can be demonstrated and learnt across all disciplines and areas. Indeed, seeing these skills and approaches in action at every contact, in every context, reinforces their importance and promotes the development of these standards of care. Healthcare professionals can all teach and continue to learn and develop these values and practices and, by so doing, ensure they are embedded in healthcare practice, staff and student education.

Continuing with radiography as an example, the following exercise can be used to help identify some of the shared skills and core proficiencies discussed above, and used as preparation for identifying IPL opportunities in a range of settings.

✐ ACTIVITY 4.12

As a practice supervisor, ask the learner to observe a patient interaction. Observe the communication styles and skills and consider how these affect the patient and/or their family. Question the learner on their understanding of the situation or to what extent the goal of the interaction was achieved. It would be ideal to carry out this exercise focusing on different IDT members. An answer guide is provided at the end of the chapter.

✐ ACTIVITY 4.13

Consider a time when you have either learned or better understood a new clinical skill through spending time with another professional. How have you been able to use this to improve your practice or education? Has this changed your understanding of their professional role?
This is a personal reflective activity, so no answer guide is provided.

It is beyond the remit of this book to detail each profession's breadth of skills and range of knowledge and procedures, but profession-specific standards can perhaps be used by practice supervisors and assessors to select delivery of procedure or skill education from the most relevant professional for students. Alternatively, with some preparation about the role of the particular professional, the student can identify these opportunities for learning when spending time with other professionals.

The example below provides detail about the amount of information that might be useful for a student to prepare prior to spending time with an AHP or other healthcare professional in order to optimise their learning and this forthcoming experience. In this example, we again return to the field of radiography. This type of information could be included within the student induction package or educational audit document so that everyone (including the students) is making their expectations clear about preparatory reading or knowledge that students require prior to attending the placement.

Background knowledge Radiographers are AHPs who are registered with the Health and Care Professions Council (HCPC). Radiographers work within a larger IDT comprising support workers, assistant practitioners, nurses, radiologists, oncologists and medical physicists. Similar to nurses, within the UK, radiographers can progress from a newly qualified band

5 radiographer into advanced practice, management and consultant roles in many specific areas or services. Radiography as a profession is split into two distinctly different areas, usually classified as either therapeutic or diagnostic. For more information you might want to refer to the following: www.sor.org/about-radiography/what-radiography-who-are-radiographers.

Radiography is required in the diagnosis, intervention and monitoring of many pathologies and injuries, hence the radiographer interacts with many other teams and with nurses across multiple specialties. Outside of the radiology department, diagnostic radiographers may visit other areas of the hospital with portable machines; such as in theatres for intraoperative imaging, or by the patient's bedside if their condition is too unstable for the safe transfer to the radiology department.

You may encounter radiographers undertaking roles such as fluoroscopy (whereby the patient's swallowing is assessed using an oral solution that is visible in real time X-ray imaging), or producing formal reports from imaging and contributing this information in IDT meetings.

The safety of patients and staff is paramount to any aspect of healthcare, but specifically within radiology where there is a legal duty to protect everyone from unintended exposure to ionising radiation. When visiting the radiology departments, the radiographer will ensure that radiation protection regulations are met by requesting that visitors remain outside the room, or stand behind a protective screen or demarcated area, or wear a lead rubber apron and possibly a thyroid guard as required. For female staff and visitors, the radiographer may enquire regarding pregnancy status to ensure that the optimum protection and guidance is provided.

ACTIVITY 4.14

Reflect on your own experiences – have you ever been a patient in a radiology department, or attended with a patient or family member?

Consider how you felt. Was it a daunting experience? Did you know what to expect?

Did you receive a clear explanation before the procedure?

Did you understand why the radiographer may have asked you to stand back, or assist, wear a lead apron or perhaps wait outside? How did that make you feel?

Is there anything that could have improved your experience? After considering this, how might you better support a patient in the future when visiting radiology?

This is a personal reflective activity, so no answer guide is provided.

Scenario 4.6 provides the example of the student nurse or midwife being supervised by the radiographer. The aim is to gain an increased understanding of the role of radiographer.

 SCENARIO 4.6

Mrs Singh is a 28-year-old pregnant lady presenting unaccompanied for a CT scan of her head. She is fearful of the procedure, which contributes to the clinical symptoms of acute confusion, agitation and short-term memory loss. This causes concern for the radiographer as Mrs Singh must remain still in order to conduct the procedure safely. To comply with radiation protection, patients should remain alone in the scanner room for a short period. The radiographer must make a clinical judgement regarding the risk to the patient and unborn baby being left unattended in the scanner, versus the risk to their health if the scan is not carried out. The radiographer must also consider the manual handling approach required to move Mrs Singh safely onto the X-ray bed, an ideal opportunity for the student to integrate and demonstrate their knowledge and ability or practise a proficiency. Radiographers will try different attempts to alleviate people's anxieties, such as using blankets and pillows for comfort and secure positioning, or through verbal reassurance or the use of therapeutic touch. Mrs Singh appears to relax and settle when listening to the radiographer – distraction techniques such as communicating through the scanner microphone system may help here. The ability to utilise small talk is a useful skill and can go a long way to reassure and distract patients.

As practice supervisor, communication via 'small talk' might come easily to you, but you might want to think about encouraging the student to take on this role: What could the student talk about that is relevant and meaningful to patients, to distract and calm them? You could encourage the students to engage in conversation with the patient about their background or hobbies and interests: do they like gardening, football, travelling, as examples.

Hopefully, the above section has provided you with increased understanding of the role of the radiographer, and you were able to recognise some shared skills with your profession. After reading this background information and going through this task, the student will be better prepared for the educational time they will spend with the radiographer, enabling them to identify LOs and relevant proficiencies for this IPL opportunity.

4.4.5 Recognising and utilising opportunities for shared learning

To deliver effective learning in practice, students must be given the opportunity to learn from a range of relevant people in the practice learning environment. By working closely with the practice supervisor or assessor, all health professionals can further empower students to be proactive in identifying and demonstrating the opportunities available to them in the various learning environments (NMC, 2018c). There may be times when a student specifically wants to work on a key proficiency (see *Scenario 4.7* for a practice example).

📂 SCENARIO 4.7

Amy, a nursing student, is spending time with Esme, a physiotherapist on a stroke unit. Amy has previously had numerous opportunities to practise proficiency 7.3: "use appropriate moving and handling equipment to support people with impaired mobility" (NMC, 2018a). Amy has not yet had the opportunity to practise the mobility aid component of 7.2: "use a range of contemporary moving and handling techniques and mobility aids". Amy is keen to utilise this opportunity during her time on the ward with Esme and discusses this with Esme. They see several complex stroke patients together with a broad range of movement difficulties. Esme explains why particular positioning techniques, equipment and aids are used, based on the needs of each patient. Not only does Amy have multiple opportunities to practise proficiency 7.2, but also, on completing her time with Esme, she reflects that in addition to this, her understanding of proficiency 7.3 is significantly enhanced. For example, Amy was not previously aware that following a stroke, a person can have an unstable shoulder joint and appropriate positioning can help prevent pain and further instability.

The example above will be used to further explore opportunities for shared learning in practice. Esme and Amy treat Jack together but have difficulty engaging him in physiotherapy due to his impaired communication. Gwen, the speech and language therapist (SLT) on the ward, carries out a joint session with them, using specialist communication techniques and aids to improve Jack's ability to understand and engage with the session. During their professional discussion, Esme and Gwen share their knowledge to identify optimal positioning for Jack considering his mobility, chest care and communication needs. During this conversation, Amy is able to bring in her knowledge about pressure care as she has recently been studying this at university and has completed a specialist placement in a community setting where this knowledge was frequently used. Not only does Jack's (and other future patients') treatment improve through this shared working, but Amy, Esme and Gwen all gain further insight into each other's professions and further knowledge regarding specific proficiencies and skills.

Notably, the success of this teamwork practice example relies on an individual's preparation, professional knowledge and skills and an understanding of different professional roles. Additionally, a willingness to remove protected boundaries and roles, factors recognised as being essential for effective IP working (Atwal, 2018), must be present. Moreover, improving Jack's care (and the care of future patients) is at the heart of this IP interaction.

D'Amour and Oandasan (2005) introduced the concept of 'interprofessionality', defined as the development of a cohesive practice between professionals from different disciplines. It is the process by which professionals reflect on and develop ways of practice that provide an integrated and cohesive answer to the needs of the client/family/population. They suggest that interprofessionality requires a paradigm shift, since IP practice has unique characteristics in terms of values, codes of conduct and ways of working. Perhaps IPL and IDT working should begin during student education to help embed these into practice. This would reduce the need for a shift in thinking, as this would become a more inherent approach to practice and delivering optimal patient care. The example used in *Scenario 4.7* also illustrates good practice, reflected in the NMC platforms 5.4, 6.2 and 6.12 (NMC, 2018a), which advise that learning culture should be transparent and foster good relations, embedding this into everyday education and practice. Students should be empowered through this education to become reflective lifelong learners and help contribute towards a culture where knowledge exchange and learning are part of daily practice for all staff working in healthcare. Although it is beyond the scope of this chapter to explore this, further widening and embracing this learning culture to include patients and their carers is part of the essence of person-centred and person-led healthcare.

4.5 SUMMARY

The value of working actively with other health professionals, as part of a single care team, is well embedded in discussions of effective healthcare (Finch, 2000). We know that collaborative working between professions is key to enhancing quality of care and the growing weight of evidence that 'teamwork works' is difficult to ignore (McPherson *et al.*, 2001). In a complex healthcare environment, all nursing, midwifery, AHPs and other healthcare professionals should be equipped with a rounded appreciation of the importance of IP collaboration. For this to become embedded, students need to learn from and about other professions, leading to a mutual understanding of professional systems, cultures and roles (George, 2000). To enable this, students need to be exposed to the wide variety of clinical disciplines that make up the IP team.

Historically, practice-based clinical supervision has been profession specific, although students spending time with other members of the IP team is not a particularly new idea. The NMC standards framework (NMC, 2018b), however, acknowledges the wealth of learning opportunities that IPL affords. As such, IPL in everyday practice could be, and arguably should be, captured more formally.

Finch (2000) urges us to think laterally around student placement experience. It is suggested that IPL taking place in the clinical setting enables the student to experience first-hand the contributions of the different team members, so embedding the philosophy of working together towards a desired goal. This is strongly in agreement with Brandt (2018) who in "a call to action for Health Professions educators" highlights that IPL offers an untapped opportunity for intentional learning and change (Nisbet *et al.*, 2013).

It is important to acknowledge, however, that the potential barriers to IPL within healthcare are considerable. Recognising the challenges is the first step in working towards solutions to overcome them. These are not insurmountable, but will require some resourcefulness on the part of AHPs as to how IPL is approached within their particular locality. Rather than viewing IPL as a burden on our time, or indeed a threat, we must remember that IPL is a multidirectional process, with AHP students being afforded similar learning opportunities to our nursing and midwifery colleagues.

A culture of openness and creativity needs to be perpetuated throughout, with AHPs advocating for the opportunities IPL brings. How the concept of IPL is interpreted will differ between localities and within clinical contexts. To allay fears and anxieties that may well build around IP supervision, we first need to define exactly what is expected. Those involved need to work closely together to contextualise IPL to the individual professional, clinical environment and higher education institution requirements. To minimise the perceived burden of IPL, and to ensure a positive learning experience for all, will require careful consideration.

As discussed previously, we know that ineffective IP collaboration can adversely affect the delivery of health services and patient care. Therefore, interventions that address issues with IP collaboration have the potential to improve professional practice and healthcare outcomes (Reeves *et al.*, 2017). One such intervention is for IP collaboration to become more embedded within the core values of nursing, midwifery and AHP students, through IPL. Having an opportunity to work alongside and learn from other healthcare professionals can surely no longer be seen as an optional extra, but should become standard practice throughout practice-based learning. Embracing the formalisation of the role of the AHP in supervising nursing and midwifery students recognises the work that has been underway for some time in this regard. Ultimately, we are all working towards the same goal of enhancing patient care. Hopefully, this chapter has addressed how this might be achieved, offering some examples that can be related to your practice.

RECOMMENDED FURTHER READING

The International Atomic Energy Agency has a useful website on ionising radiations, and radiography-specific information regarding pregnancy and radiation: https://www.iaea.org/resources/rpop/health-professionals/radiology/pregnant-women#9 (accessed 14 August 2020).

For further reading on safety in magnetic resonance imaging: www.sor.org/learning/document-library/safety-magnetic-resonance-imaging-0 (accessed 14 August 2020).

REFERENCES

Atwal, A. (2018) Interprofessional learning interventions: championing a lost cause? *Evidence-Based Nursing*, **21**: 32–3.

Belinsky, S.B. and Tataronis, G.R. (2007) Past experiences of the clinical instructor and current attitudes toward evaluation of students. *Journal of Allied Health*, **36**(1): 11–16.

Brandt, F.B. (2018) Rethinking health professions education through the lens of interprofessional practice and education. *New Directions for Adult and Continuing Education*, **157**: 65–76. doi: 10.1002/ace.20269

Bynum, W.E. and Haque, T.M. (2016) Risky business: psychological safety and the risks of learning medicine. *Journal of Graduate Medical Education*, **8**(5): 780–2.

Centre for the Advancement of Interprofessional Education (2019) *About CAIPE*. CAIPE. Available at: www.caipe.org/about-us (accessed 14 August 2020).

Cruess, S.R., Cruess, R.L. and Steinert, Y. (2008) Role modelling – making the most of a powerful teaching strategy. *British Medical Journal*, **29**(336):7646: 718–21.

D'Amour, D. and Oandasan, I. (2005) Interprofessionality as the field of interprofessional practice and interprofessional education: An emerging concept. *Journal of Interprofessional Care*, **19(Suppl 1):** 8–20. doi: 10.1080/13561820500081604

Davis, J. (2013) Modelling as a strategy for learning and teaching in nursing education. *Singapore Nursing Journal*, **40(3):** 5–10.

Department of Health (2001) *Working together – learning together: a framework for lifelong learning for the NHS*. Department of Health.

Department of Health (2002) *Learning from Bristol: the Department of Health's response to the report of the public inquiry into children's heart surgery at the Bristol Royal Infirmary 1984–1995*. Department of Health.

Department of Health/CAIPE (2007) *Creating an interprofessional workforce: an education and training framework for health and social care in England*. Department of Health.

Department of Health and Social Care (2019) *NHS long term plan*. Department of Health and Social Care

Donaldson, J.H. and Carter, D. (2005) The value of role modelling: Perceptions of undergraduate and diploma nursing (adult) students. *Nurse Education in Practice*, **5:** 353–9.

Emerson, T. (2004) Preparing placement supervisors for primary care: an interprofessional perspective from the UK. *Journal of Interprofessional Care*, **18(2):** 165–82.

Finch, J. (2000) Interprofessional education and teamworking: a view from the education providers. *British Medical Journal*, **321:** 1138–40.

Fisher, M. and Kiernan, M. (2019) Student nurses' lived experience of patient safety and raising concerns. *Nurse Education Today*, **77:** 1–5.

Flynn, S. (2011) Role model. In: McIntosh-Scott, A., Gidman, J. and Mason-Whitehead, E. (editors) *Key concepts in health education*. Sage.

Francis, R. (2013) *Report of the Mid-Staffordshire NHS Foundation Trust Public Inquiry Executive Summary*. The Stationery Office.

George, C. (2000) *Teamworking in medicine*. General Medical Council.

Gilligan, C., Outram, S. and Levett-Jones, T. (2014) Recommendations from recent graduates in medicine, nursing and pharmacy on improving interprofessional education in university programs: a qualitative study. *BMC Medical Education*, **14:** 52. doi: 10.1186/1472-6920-14-52

Health and Care Professions Council (2011) *Professionalism in healthcare professionals – research report*. Available at: www.hcpc-uk.org/resources/reports/2011/professionalism-in-healthcare-professionals/ (accessed 14 August 2020).

Health and Care Professions Council (2018) *Standards of education and training.* Available at: www.hcpc-uk.org/standards/standards-relevant-to-education-and-training/set/ (accessed 14 August 2020).

Hinton, J. (2014) The application of role models in health education. *Operating Department Practice Journal*, 2(4): 194–200.

Hood, K., Cant, R., Leech, M., Baulch, J. and Gilbee, A. (2014) Trying on the professional self: nursing students' perceptions of learning about roles, identity and teamwork in an interprofessional clinical placement. *Applied Nursing Research*, 27: 109–14.

Interprofessional Education Collaborative Expert Panel (2011) *Core competencies for interprofessional collaborative practice: Report of an expert panel.* Interprofessional Education Collaborative. Available at: www.pcpcc.org/sites/default/files/resources/Core%20Competencies%20for%20Interprofessional%20Collaborative%20Practice.pdf (accessed 14 August 2020).

Jack, K., Hamshire, C., Harris, W.E. *et al.* (2018) "My mentor didn't speak to me for the first four weeks": Perceived unfairness experienced by nursing students in clinical practice settings. *Journal of Clinical Nursing*, 27(5–6): 929–38. doi: 10.1111/jocn.14015

Jackson, M., Pelone, F., Reeves, S. *et al.* (2016) Interprofessional education in the care of people diagnosed with dementia and their carers: a systematic review. *BMJ Open*, 6(8). doi: 10.1136/bmjopen-2015-010948

Johnson, J.A. (2015) Nursing professional development specialists as role models. *Journal for Nurses in Professional Development*, 31(5): 297–9.

Levett-Jones, T. and Lathlean, J. (2009a) The ascent to competence conceptual framework: An outcome of a study of belongingness. *Journal of Clinical Nursing*, 18: 2870–9.

Levett-Jones, T., Lathlean, J., Higgins, I. and McMillan, M. (2009b) Staff–student relationships and their impact on nursing students' belongingness and learning. *Journal of Advanced Nursing*, 65(2): 316–24.

McPherson, K., Headrick, L. and Moss, F. (2001) Working and learning together: good quality care depends on it, but how can we achieve it? *Quality in Health Care*, 10: 46–53.

Morison, S., Boohan, M., Jenkins, J. and Moutray, M. (2003) Facilitating undergraduate interprofessional learning in healthcare: comparing classroom and clinical learning for nursing and medical students. *Learning in Health and Social Care*, 2(2): 92–104.

Nancarrow, S.A., Booth, A., Ariss, S. *et al.* (2013) Ten principles of good interdisciplinary team work. *Human Resources for Health*, **11(1)**: 19.

Nisbet, G., Lincoln, M. and Dunn, S. (2013) Informal interprofessional learning: An untapped opportunity for learning and change within the workplace. *Journal of Interprofessional Care*, **27(6)**: 469–75.

Nursing and Midwifery Council (2018a) *Future nurse: Standards of proficiency for registered nurses.* NMC. Available at <u>www.nmc.org.uk/globalassets/sitedocuments/education-standards/future-nurse-proficiencies.pdf</u> (accessed 13 August 2020).

Nursing and Midwifery Council (2018b) *Realising professionalism: Part 1: Standards framework for nursing and midwifery education.* NMC. Available at: <u>www.nmc.org.uk/globalassets/sitedocuments/education-standards/education-framework.pdf</u> (accessed 13 August 2020).

Nursing and Midwifery Council (2018c) *Realising professionalism: Part 2: Standards for student supervision and assessment.* NMC. Available at: <u>www.nmc.org.uk/globalassets/sitedocuments/education-standards/student-supervision-assessment.pdf</u> (accessed 13 August 2020).

Nursing and Midwifery Council (2018d) *Standards of proficiency for nursing associates.* NMC. Available at: <u>www.nmc.org.uk/globalassets/sitedocuments/education-standards/nursing-associates-proficiency-standards.pdf</u> (accessed 14 August 2020).

Nursing and Midwifery Council (2019) *Different learning opportunities.* NMC. Available at: <u>www.nmc.org.uk/supporting-information-on-standards-for-student-supervision-and-assessment/learning-environments-and-experiences/types-of-learning-experiences/different-learning-opportunities/</u> (accessed 14 August 2020).

Oandasan, I. and Reeves, S. (2005) Key elements for interprofessional education. Part 1: The learner, the educator and the learning context. *Journal of Interprofessional Care*, **19(Suppl 1)**: 21–38.

Overton, A., Clark, M. and Thomas, Y. (2009) A review of non-traditional occupational therapy practice placement education: a focus on role-emerging and project placements. *British Journal of Occupational Therapy*, **72(7)**: 294–301.

Palese, A., Gonella, S., Brugnolli, A. *et al.* (2019) Nursing students' interprofessional educational experiences in the clinical context: findings from an Italian cross-sectional study. *BMJ Open*, **9(3)**. doi: 10.1136/bmjopen-2018-025575

Reeves, S., Fletcher, S., Barr, H. *et al.* (2016) A BEME systematic review of the effects of interprofessional education: BEME Guide no. 39. *Medical Teacher*, **38(7)**: 656–8. doi: 10.3109/0142159X.2016.1173663

Reeves, S., Pelone, F., Harrison, R., Goldman, J. and Zwarenstein, M. (2017) Interprofessional collaboration to improve professional practice and healthcare outcomes. *Cochrane Database of Systematic Reviews*, 6(6). doi:10.1002/14651858.CD000072.pub3

Reeves, S., Perrier, L., Goldman, J., Freeth, D. and Zwarenstein, M. (2013) Interprofessional education: Effects on professional practice and healthcare outcomes. *Cochrane Database of Systematic Reviews*, 3. doi: 10.1002/14651858.CD002213.pub3

ACTIVITY ANSWER GUIDES

ACTIVITY 4.5

You may have thought of the following questions or conversations to have:
* What year of nurse/midwifery education is Jenny in? How much clinical experience has she had so far?
* What learning outcomes (LOs) is she hoping to achieve during her time with you?
* What are your and Jenny's expectations for the time that you are to spend together? How much will Jenny be able to contribute? Will there be time for discussion and reflection?
* What does Jenny, as a learner, understand about your profession and role? What do you know about the AHP role?
* How does she feel this experience links with her own future profession?

The person responsible for coordinating a student such as Jenny's learning may have developed a plan for the placement and updated you on the LOs the student wishes to achieve with you. Therefore, you may already have directed the student to read around topics related to your role. By establishing an open and inclusive environment, the student can focus on learning and achieving their learning outcomes.

ACTIVITY 4.6

Various options could help Jenny achieve this outcome. She could liaise with several health professionals to learn more about this topic, such as:
* The pharmacist may feel the best approach to share knowledge is through an informal teaching session away from the ward, discussing types of pain relief and indications for use in certain patient types

- The physiotherapist may prefer direct patient contact and demonstrate how careful positioning of a patient in a bed or a chair may relieve pain and discomfort
- The OT may demonstrate how adjusting the height of beds and chairs may reduce pain and discomfort; this may be through direct patient contact or away from the ward looking at the range of equipment that may be available.

ACTIVITY 4.8

How does Anila make David feel at ease?

She acquires knowledge of the programme that David is studying. She asks David about his previous experience, knowledge and skills. She acknowledges any fears or anxieties that David might have. Anila uses a range of communication techniques and active listening skills to understand David's learning requirements. Anila ensures that David can observe, rehearse and practise and engage in the real work of the ward or unit. David needs to feel like he 'belongs' in order to learn.

ACTIVITY 4.12

Let us consider this activity with a radiographer and their patient. Upon meeting the patient, the radiographer will ask a set of patient identification questions to satisfy the radiation regulations. This provides an ideal opportunity to assess the patient, providing insight into cognitive and sensory ability, which may inform the radiographer on how they adapt their technique to the individual. Often the radiographer will use verbal and non-verbal cues in investigation of the patient's clothing, by asking questions or checking clothing and pockets to feel for any clips or adjusters on undergarments, or for the presence of other items such as reading glasses. When asking the patient to "breathe in and hold", required for a chest X-ray, often the radiographer will verbally communicate the command, while demonstrating the action. This can be followed by asking the patient to demonstrate their understanding to ensure the procedure is effective. This specific example helps to identify just some of the shared skills and core proficiencies discussed above, highlighting the many varied and diverse opportunities for IPL in clinical practice.

Let us now return to the answers generated by the activity regarding identified differences in knowledge and skills required between professions, alongside referring to the nursing standards of proficiency to further consider differences between professions. Annexe B describes a broad range of procedures and skills specific to nursing such as: "2.10: Measure and interpret blood glucose levels". Similar standards of proficiency are in place for 16 healthcare professions under the auspices of the health and care professions council (www.hcpc-uk.org/standards/standards-of-proficiency). These provide detail of procedures and skills specific to each profession such as: "13.10: Understand the principles behind the use of nutritional analysis programs to analyse food intake records and recipes and interpret the results" from the standards of proficiency for dietetics.

CHAPTER 5

FACILITATING LEARNING THROUGH FEEDBACK AND FEEDFORWARD

Peggy Murphy and Hannah Dixon

5.1 INTRODUCTION

Earlier in this book in *Chapter 3* we outlined some ideas about providing students with feedback as part of the repertoire of the clinical supervisor and assessor. This chapter provides more detail and practical advice in order to equip you with a broader range of approaches to provide feedback and, perhaps more importantly, feedforward information for learners. Feedforward techniques have gained increasing importance as we have come to understand that students require information delivered in a particular manner in order to help them to develop and learn, by applying techniques and advice to future practice.

After reading this chapter you will be able to:
- Discuss a range of feedback and feedforward techniques
- Apply these techniques to a range of situations that you might face in your role as a practice supervisor or assessor.

5.2 WHAT IS FEEDBACK IN CLINICAL PRACTICE?

Feedback is any material that advises us how we are doing in relation to meeting our goals. It is information that can be used to improve performance. For feedback to be effective it needs to highlight what the learner has done well and what the learner needs to improve (Murphy and Morley, 2020). When feedback is offered in a constructive way it can be very powerful and enhance student learning. Hounsell (2004) develops this idea, explaining that feedback is any information, process or activity which affords accelerated learning. This definition of feedback identifies that students can self-assess and that they often give themselves feedback according to how well they think they are doing. In other words, they consider how well they measure up to any task. Self-assessment and feedback are skills to be encouraged in all practitioners and self-appraisal is integral to any professional role (see *Chapter 7* for further discussion).

Feedback is more than simply measuring performance and marking it; it can also be used as a distinct learning tool. Anyone with an educational role in practice will be aware of the necessity to make final judgements on the student's ability to perform against professional body criteria. To do that successfully educators need to be cognisant of a student's learning level and (prior to passing that final judgement on a student's ability to perform and undertake a task) they need to be aware that there are a myriad of opportunities to use feedback to promote students' learning. When creating learning opportunities and 'mock' or formative assessments, it is also important to acknowledge that feedback is not a one-way process from the educator to the students. It is the starting point of a conversation about learning. While it is true that students themselves will pass or fail a placement, educators have an essential role in preparing students to learn and develop. Practice supervisors are in a unique position to provide feedback opportunities that impact upon a student's learning in placement. Indeed, this feedback, when acted upon by the student, can support a subsequent positive summative assessment undertaken by the practice assessor.

5.3 WHAT IS FEEDFORWARD IN CLINICAL PRACTICE?

When practice supervisors offer feedforward, students have the opportunity to adapt their work. They can utilise feedback from self-appraisal and feedback from others prior to being finally assessed by the practice assessor. As feedforward happens prior to the final assessment, it creates a formative assessment opportunity. The concept of feedforward is vitally important as a learning tool to ensure that practice supervisors and assessors offer students as many opportunities as possible to develop their skills. Students who are proactive and engage with this approach are more likely to reflect upon feedback in a way that helps them to design strategies for their own learning success (Murphy and Morley, 2020). A practice supervisor's role is to support students in practice and to help them make the connections between assessment, feedback and learning.

The student journey is a formative experience and students are continuously being asked to learn new skills, knowledge and competencies. To promote successful learning in practice, students need to take responsibility for their own learning. While they are developing, they may require a 'guide on the side' to help them to make sense of all the new information and feedback they are given. Not all students know what to do with feedback and assisting them through the process enables students to use feedback effectively so they can develop into competent practitioners. It is often those in most need of feedback that have the least idea of what to do with it. Using formative assessments and spending time discussing feedback, as well as the importance of feedback for the student's personal and professional development, can help students to become empowered and independent lifelong learners. Nicol and Macfarlane-Dick (2006) suggest that this process helps students to take control over their own learning. As a practice supervisor you can assist students to make sense of feedback so they can use it to develop and scaffold onto their existing knowledge. Indeed, the use of Socratic questioning techniques introduced to you in *Chapter 3* can be used to support the feedback process.

5.4 THE PRINCIPLES OF EFFECTIVE FEEDBACK

Good feedback lets the student know what they are doing well, as well as what they could improve (Nicol and Macfarlane-Dick, 2006). When giving feedback to students in order to help them make sense it is important to offer specific examples. For example, if you have seen a student struggle with initiating a conversation with patients or encourage interaction, rather than giving generalised feedback saying "You need to improve your communication skills", it may be beneficial to ask the student how they think they could convey more warmth and encourage interaction with patients. You may think students do not require guidance on something so simple as introducing themselves but it is not just students who need reminding about this. They may need your advice on many aspects of communication. For example, when giving specific advice on how to initiate a conversation you could suggest "Hello my name is" as a start. This approach was highlighted in a campaign by Dr Kate Granger after she was hospitalised herself. She noted that many staff did not introduce themselves before delivering care to her and decided to start a campaign. For more information see: www.hellomynameis.org.uk/

Although introductions may seem extremely obvious to you as an experienced nurse or midwife and practice supervisor, introductions may not come naturally to a student. Students often feel overwhelmed by 'information overload' when trying to remember everything on placement so that they then forget the basics. When giving feedback it is useful to think that students often require simple explanations supported by examples of 'good performance'. Sometimes educators need to show students what they want rather than tell them. If you can offer specific examples about what is required it makes it easier for students to understand the standard they need to perform to.

According to Nicol and Macfarlane-Dick (2006, p. 205) there are seven principles of good feedback practice. These principles can be applied by the practice supervisor and practice assessor:

1. Helps clarify what good performance is (goals, criteria, expected standards)
2. Facilitates the development of self-assessment (reflection) in learning
3. Delivers high-quality information to students about their learning
4. Encourages teacher and peer dialogue around learning
5. Encourages positive motivational beliefs and self-esteem
6. Provides opportunities to close the gap between current and desired performance
7. Provides information to teachers that can be used to help shape teaching.

A simple way to give structure and guidance on the principles of giving and receiving effective feedback and reinforcement that effective feedback is a gift for learning is to use the acronym GIFT (*Table 5.1*).

Table 5.1: GIFT: a framework for effective feedback

Generosity	Giving developmental (or formative) feedback is recognised as one of the most important interactions in a learning environment and a fundamental building block (Race, 2014). Highlighting that feedback is a gift for learning needs to be communicated between both student and educator. This can be done with the spirit of generosity rather than one of reproach. Try to introduce the importance of working with feedback early on in the student/educator relationship. Offer it as a gift for students to reflect upon. Highlighting the reflective element enables students to develop their own work following feedback, rather than simply seeing it as criticism (Winstone *et al.*, 2017). Giving effective feedback is a gift as it demonstrates that you care sufficiently about developing the work of another to observe, reflect and offer advice on their work in a way that supports their learning (Brookhart, 2017). In your role as practice supervisor it is critical that you help students view feedback as an opportunity for growth.
Interactive	Educators need to explore ways to develop students to become active users of feedback. Not all students understand the importance of feedback in relation to learning or professional development. One strategy is to introduce the concept of feedback as a tool for learning during induction or at your first meeting with students. There are a number of ways to encourage interaction, and one is to role model working with feedback. You could demonstrate to students any feedback you have received and show the action plan you constructed as a result of

Table 5.1: (cont'd)

	that feedback from others. This could be feedback you have gathered for the NMC revalidation, for example. This sets a scene to the student that all nurses need to work with feedback. Remember that feedback is most effective when it is given as soon as possible following the activity being assessed. Timely feedback helps students focus and reflect on their actions to become more self-regulated learners. Another way is to ask students what area of their practice they would like feedback on.
Feedforward	Feedforward is a term used for comments that enable students to improve their future work. Feedforward empowers students by giving them an opportunity to adapt their work by using feedback before a final judgement (or summative assessment) is made. Practice supervisors can create opportunities for students to learn about skills, knowledge and competency and give feedback (as feedforward) so students have an opportunity to reflect and amend their practice before being summatively assessed. Creating 'mock assessments' is one method through which practice supervisors and assessors can create learning opportunities. Communication is often fraught with complication and what you think you have said is not necessarily what the other hears or understands. Students need opportunities to check what you have meant by the feedback you offered to them and then apply what they have learned from feedback in the practice setting. As a practice supervisor when you give feedforward you are giving students a real chance to learn, amend their behaviour and develop as a professional.
Trigger	There are two triggers. The first trigger is a trigger for action. Feedback should not be viewed as 'fixed' but as 'a dynamic process' that enhances performance. Students may require some help in writing action plans based on the feedback they receive; making sure they are involved makes this process more developmental and less punitive. As such, feedback needs to be offered in a way that facilitates change. Students often require guidance to understand how feedback enables them to become active reflectors in order for them to improve *their* work. There is an emotional dimension to the teacher/learner relationship and it is important that both adopt an emotional state that is conducive to learning by viewing feedback as part of conversation (Mortiboys, 2012; Nicol, 2010). This trigger is more likely to have a positive effect if practice supervisors encourage students to question how feedback helps them to achieve their overall aims and objectives in placement. The second trigger is acknowledging that feedback can cause an emotional response. Receiving feedback can challenge a student's emotions. All feedback needs to be given in a sensitive manner. Acknowledging that there is likely to be an emotional reaction helps students notice feedback triggers in them. Practice supervisors can plan around the fact that there will be emotional responses to their feedback and can build in 'touch points' to create dialogue with students following feedback. Often students need a little time to regulate their emotions following feedback so it can be useful to allow students time to reflect upon comments before discussing their reactions to feedback. This time to reflect can vary from student to student but having a conversation about how the feedback made them feel directly after feedback is not always appropriate and sometimes it is better to leave a little space before discussing ways they can manage emotional responses. Practice supervisors can facilitate students developing emotional intelligence when working with feedback and help students consider what actions they need to take to manage their emotional responses.

5.5 FEEDBACK FOR LEARNING

Feedback is part of the learning cycle. The potential for offering good feedback is that it gives students access to information about their performance. This in turn allows them some sense of control to develop their own work. Not all students work well with feedback and there may be a variety of reasons for this. One reason may be that they do not believe they can improve. It is part of a practice supervisor's role to support student learning, so they gain confidence and build their skills in practice. Learning is more than the acquisition of knowledge from an expert transmitting their knowledge and skills to another. Learning is unlikely to occur by 'downloading' information from one person's memory bank into another's. All of us are more likely to learn by interacting with knowledge and skills in order to make sense and meaning from the experience. Some students do not have a lot of belief in their ability to learn.

Part of the human learning experience is learning through play, mistakes and error. Most of us learn to walk by coming to terms with falling down numerous times but that does not deter us from working towards our goal. The fear of falling (and failing) does not stop us from trying again. Some students forget this and can become almost paralysed with fear about getting things wrong. When students have a 'fixed mindset' they fear that they cannot improve due to a lack of innate ability, and this can hamper their progress. Students can be introduced to the concept of growth mindset (Dweck, 2011). Developing a growth mindset, or feedback mindset, enables students to view challenges as opportunities to learn from. Not all learning is comfortable and sometimes learning involves failure. Creating a learning environment where students are sufficiently nurtured so that they feel safe, while encouraging them to push out of their comfort zones, is complex. Even an experienced practice supervisor can make a wrong decision as to whether a student is ready or not to be nudged into their next stage of development.

Working in partnership with students and enabling them to take some control over their own learning in these circumstances can help them to develop problem-solving skills and the ability to solve problems is a key attribute in nursing.

> ☰ **TOP TIP**
>
> Applying the definition of coaching introduced to you in *Chapter 3* can support a positive feedback mindset that starts students in a process whereby they can value themselves as change agents in control over their own learning rather than passive recipients of someone else's judgement. Coaching in *Chapter 3* is defined as an approach adopted by supervisors and assessors that facilitates the student's learning and development and this is achieved through unlocking the student's own potential.

There is no single learning experience or approach that would enable every student to make sense of *all* of their learning. As a practice supervisor you will develop your own strategies to meet the learning needs of a variety of students. It is important to understand underpinning principles of learning and teaching. One such approach proposed by Healey *et al.* (2014) is the student engagement framework 'students as partners'. This framework advocates the requirement for honesty, inclusive empowerment and trust. This method suggests that students are more than customers, and advocates using a partnership approach to teaching, learning and assessment. The 'students as partners' approach takes both staff and students outside of their comfort zone and there is a significant shift in power. Power is shared and this can lead to uncertain outcomes. The Nursing and Midwifery Council (NMC, 2018a) has stressed the importance of student empowerment and it is integral to the new standards for education and training. It highlights that student empowerment is required to achieve the required proficiencies in practice and also recognises that empowerment leads to power sharing. One way to encourage students to take control and become independent lifelong learners is to enable them to assess their own work. Teaching self-assessment takes a lot of skill and patience and requires the practice supervisor to take a step back and consider their role in the education of students. Education is not simply about teaching content to students so they know 'stuff'. Teaching empowerment involves sharing information and experiences with students so that they can grasp the fundamental principles of independent lifelong learning. This takes time and effort and sometimes a leap of faith.

Courage is required from both the teacher and the student in order to enable such a transformative relationship. It also involves a recognition that both will learn throughout the process. Discussing expectations in the introductory meeting at the start of the placement of both parties is essential to forming a reciprocal relationship of trust. Informing the students that they will be both giving and receiving feedback throughout the partnership is essential. Once students understand the rationale for feedback it helps them to make sense of it in relation to their personal and professional development. This can be made evident in relation to giving effective person-centred care or in relation to any particular competency that the student is being assessed on for their learning portfolio. Once students understand the purpose of feedback it can lead to engaging with it to improve their performance.

ACTIVITY 5.1

Consider the following questions:
- How often do you receive feedback as a practitioner?
- How often would you like to receive feedback in your role and what elements would you like feedback on?
- Who gives you feedback?
- Do you ask for feedback and, if so, what are the most effective ways to do this?
- When you receive feedback how does it make you feel?
- Are there skills to be developed in how to give and receive feedback and, if so, what are they?
- What circumstances are likely to be the catalyst for you receiving feedback?

An answer guide is provided at the end of the chapter.

5.6 THE FEEDBACK CONVERSATION: FEEDBACK AS A RECIPROCAL PROCESS

Day (2019) suggests that effective feedback happens when there is a concerted effort to create a learning culture that fosters feedback. Working with students involves constantly giving and receiving feedback. Giving feedback is not a one-way process. Students need to have the opportunity to engage with *their* feedback by questioning what it means to *their* practice and performance, otherwise a learning opportunity could be lost (Day, 2019). Working with students so they understand takes patience and courage. Whenever you hold a feedback conversation this creates an opportunity to establish which comments students find useful and why. This is useful information to you as an educator and to the student so they can take the information to other placement areas (Wilson, 2019). There are some suggestions about holding difficult conversations later in this chapter. Good feedback involves dialogue and there are a number of questions that students can ask to help them to probe practice supervisors so they can elicit useful feedback. It would be useful to again refer to *Chapter 3* where questioning is explored in detail.

5.6.1 *Power and emotion associated with feedback*

Occasionally you will have conversations whereby you have given feedback to a student and will consider that you have given full guidance on all the issues that the student needs to address in order to be successful on placement. The student will passively appear to have understood. It is when practice supervisors and assessors are having feedback conversations that Wilson (2019) suggests they acknowledge 'two elephants in the room'. Those two elephants are emotion and power. She suggests that educators need to give students permission to be upset during the dialogue. This can be facilitated by opening up feedback with coaching conversations and inviting students to say how they feel about receiving feedback. Wilson (2019) advocates initiating feedback conversations by shifting the emphasis from the educator telling someone where they went wrong to a more mutual position of 'let's work this out together'. She encourages conversations about how students think they can improve themselves and eliciting whether they understand the meaning behind any feedback for improvement. Working in partnership with students enables a two-way dialogue. Partnership working in any context involves an exploration of who holds the power; therefore it is essential to leave spaces or pauses in a feedback conversation to avoid it being a monologue, so as to encourage a two-way conversation. Students need to make sense of feedback and learn to engage with feedback. Those individuals responsible for learning in the practice environment should consider ways to encourage students to be more independent learners and less dependent on another's judgement.

It would be useful to think back to *Chapter 3* where you were introduced to the work of Scott's work around 'radical candour' where the emphasis is placed on the practice supervisor and practice assessor offering direct and honest (constructive) and genuine feedback (Scott, 2017).

5.7 PROFESSIONAL REQUIREMENTS FOR FEEDBACK

The NMC explicitly refers to the professional values enshrined within giving and receiving feedback in Section 9.1 of *The Code* (NMC, 2018c). Working with feedback is a large part of the revalidation process. Revalidation asks registrants to demonstrate that they have actively sought

ACTIVITY 5.2

Tea and biscuit assessment criteria

This activity is designed to prepare you to give feedback to students by taking a routine activity and thinking about how the use of feedback could enhance performance. It involves you considering how to make a mid-morning snack for your peer. You have to take into consideration how you will meet your peer's personal standards and whether their drink is served with or without food (such as a biscuit).

Task 1 Consider three standards or requirements that need to be met in order for another person to make your mid-morning snack to your satisfaction. Here are some examples:

Hot drinks have to be piping hot
Tea must be served by putting the milk in first (or last)
Teabag must be removed
Tea must be served in a china cup.

If you are not particularly fussy, make up some 'standards' based upon other people's requirements. Write these down and do not show the other person. You can discuss these requirements verbally.

Task 2 You may also want to think about how these standards would be partially met or completely met, or not met at all.

Task 3 Talk to your peer and establish exactly how they take their tea/coffee/cold drink – consider what cup/glass/plate you will serve them with. Change places so each of you has explored what the other wants as a mid-morning snack.

Task 4 Both you and your peer need to *individually* create two tweets of 180 characters or less to describe how both your and their mid-morning snack should be made.

Task 5 Return to your pairs and consider both tweets on a scale of 1–10. Assess your partner's tweet and state how near to your original standards your partner has achieved. If they have not scored 10 (the highest score) how could you advise them to improve to meet your standard? If they have scored 10 how can you give feedback to them so they can build on this skill in the future?

Finally, consider how you felt following the feedback that your partner gave you about this exercise and whether it would enable you to make them a better mid-morning snack.

This is a personal reflective activity, so no answer guide is provided.

out, reflected and acted upon feedback on their practice. The revalidation requires nurses to submit five pieces of practice-related feedback. The underpinning thought is that nurses need to seek advice about how they are performing in work. The NMC also gives more specific advice in the new standards for education and training about how giving and receiving feedback is essential to practice supervision. Standard 3.3 (NMC, 2018b) requires practice supervisors to: "support and supervise students, providing feedback on their progress towards, and achievement of, proficiencies and skills". The standards also state that practice supervisors are required to provide feedback on students' conduct and where they think that students have not met the standard, and to assist students' ability to consider how they can improve. Practice supervisors, along with others, need to offer constructive feedback and assist students in putting together action plans that will help students improve their performance. Similar feedback is also required by the practice assessor following any summative assessment performed.

5.8 PEER FEEDBACK

The new standards for education and training (NMC, 2018a) require students to be supervisor ready at the point of registration. With this in mind, practice supervisors should provide students with opportunities to give feedback to their peers and other colleagues. It is a professional requirement from Section 9.1 of *The Code* that nurses: "provide honest, accurate and constructive feedback to colleagues" (NMC, 2018c). The ability to do this well does not happen overnight and requires practice to become proficient at it. Sambell *et al.* (2016) advocate involving students in peer assessment and feedback in order to enable them to develop skills to become self-sufficient in monitoring their own work, rather than being dependent upon someone else to assess their work for them. There is evidence to state that peer assessment enables students to become more independent learners. Providing opportunities for peer assessment and feedback enables students to be both supervisor ready and develop as lifelong learners. Engaging in peer assessment also provides opportunities for students to hone their skills of giving feedback that is both tactful and useful.

5.8.1 Helping students to develop their peer feedback techniques

Nurses work within teams to ensure that people's needs are met. Learning how to assess another professional's or peer's work while you are a student prepares you for your role in a demanding professional workforce. At the point of registration as a nurse, or soon after preceptorship in most but

ACTIVITY 5.3

Student peer assessment: ways to give constructive feedback

Facilitator action: work with two students, explaining to them the following directed learning activity:

Directed learning activity

By the end of this directed learning activity you will be able to:
- Consider how to give and receive effective feedback to enhance learning
- Consider how to transfer that knowledge to students in your placement area
- Use the acronym GRATEFUL (see *Table 5.2*) to think about how to provide peer feedback
- Use a checklist to guide the process of giving feedback.

Facilitator action: continuing on the theme of seeing feedback as a gift to learning, the guidance in *Table 5.2* uses the acronym GRATEFUL in the hope it may be helpful for those inexperienced in giving peer feedback; work through the acronym with the two students.

Facilitator action: when the students have worked through the acronym GRATEFUL, introduce the peer assessment checklist (*Table 5.3*) to them and provide the opportunity for them to complete it.

Facilitator action: reflect on the impact of this activity once completed with the student.

This is a personal reflective activity, so no answer guide is provided.

Assessing peers is adapted from the following document: https://cpd.web.ucu. org.uk/files/2013/06/CPD_factsheet_peer_review.pdf

not all areas you are likely to begin supervising students and others in your selected area of practice. Learning how to be tactful when giving feedback can improve the quality of service-user experience and (if done well) should be a positive experience for all involved.

Being able to assess your own work and the work of others is useful to creating healthy workplaces. Teamwork involves communicating and feeding back how others are performing in relation to the service goals. The Mid-Staffordshire NHS Foundation Trust Public Enquiry known as the Francis report (Francis, 2013) noted that students were well placed to observe and report on both good and poor practice and that it is essential to change the culture of healthcare and encourage practitioners to speak to each other in ways that enhance practice and ensure safe and competent care delivery. Nurses are required to be lifelong learners who need to engage throughout their careers in seeking new ways to improve the experience of the people they serve.

You may already have knowledge and experience in giving feedback to students about how they are developing their skills in practice. Think of ways in which you can utilise that knowledge to support two students to give and receive feedback to each other in the practice area. *Activity 5.3* is designed to help you develop peer learning and provides you with a resource to facilitate a directed learning activity on feedback for students in your placement area. Facilitator actions are provided that will guide you as the facilitator through the activity.

Table 5.2: GRATEFUL: a framework for providing peer feedback

Guide your peers	Suggest ways and show peers how they may improve their work. It is easier to point out shortfalls than it is to offer constructive feedback on how to put things right; however, it is essential that you adopt a supportive stance. Peer assessment should be a meaningful experience for both parties.
Reflect	This is an opportunity to develop reflective practice for growth. Reflect on the guidelines throughout any activity or assessment. Use the guidelines to direct your feedback.
Aim high	Peer assessing is a reciprocal process and can be used as a method to set, maintain or establish standards. The standard you are prepared to accept will become the standard you will work to in the future; set your standards high. When you set high expectations, you stretch yourself and your peers. Nobody can rise to a low expectation.
Timely	Feedback is more helpful when it is given in a timely fashion, preferably immediately after the assessment. Think about what you are assessing and create opportunities for two-way communication.
Empathetic	Your role as a peer assessor is to support the learning of others in your group. Put yourself in the shoes of the peer whose paper you are assessing. Only give feedback on the assessment that is set. Make sure through dialogue that you and your peer both understand what the assessment is and avoid giving feedback on anything other than your peer's work.
Focus on development	You are a resource to your peers, as they are to you. Peers can use feedback to help their personal and professional development. When your peers do well let them know – celebrate with them. Conversely if your peer's work in practice might fail, then consider if it is kinder to flag that up and give your peer a chance to reflect on and amend their work *OR* is it more professional to say nothing and wait to see if your group member fails their placement?
Understanding	If their work is not at the required standard, then you will need to be sensitive as well as honest in helping your peers achieve the required standard. Think about the kindest support you can offer as a professional in the making. Honest feedback is essential to learning, particularly when it is given to help someone improve. Demonstrate that everyone needs guidance about areas of their work and how to get better in order for them to develop as lifelong learners.
Learn	Assessing other people develops your own learning and enables you to consider the assessment process from the viewpoint of an assessor. It also gives you the opportunity to experience the level of work your peers are achieving. This can help you to assist in the development of others and raise your own performance. Peer assessment helps to create a community of practice whereby peers start to view each other as essential to learning and respect each other as a valuable resource.

Table 5.3: Peer assessment checklist

Question	Yes	No	Comment
Have I based my peer assessment on the appropriate assessment guidelines?			
Have I constructively criticised this work and expressed my comments in an honest and tactful manner?			
Have I clearly directed this peer on how to improve their work?			
Have my assessment and comments been offered in a manner that will assist my peer's learning?			
Putting myself in my peer's shoes, would I benefit from the experience I am offering?			
Will my comments help my peer develop into a more competent health and social care professional?			
What have I learned from this experience?			
What has my peer learned from this experience?			

Another way to help students interact with feedback is to suggest they create action plans to turn passive reflection into active reflection on feedback. This enables students to receive feedback, reflect upon feedback, act on feedback and then apply that feedback to similar care scenarios in practice.

To help students turn the reflective cycle (*Figure 5.1*) into manageable chunks of action they may be guided to use frameworks such as the Specific, Measurable, Achievable, Realistic and Timely: **SMART** framework. This

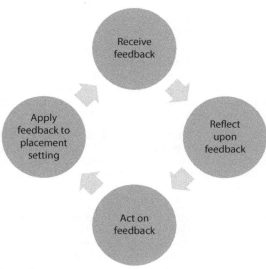

Figure 5.1: Reflective cycle.

will help them to turn feedback into action that will help their development. For example, you may have commented that the student has good verbal communication with the people in their care but that their body language does not always match this (see *Table 5.4*).

Table 5.4: Using SMART language

S	**Specifically** the student's body language does not match their verbal communication; for example, you could help the learner by stating that when you say good morning at the start of the shift you have your arms folded and that you do not often smile.
M	**Measure** their performance in this area, e.g. "I have noticed this on three consecutive shifts".
A	Suggest **achievable** goals such as greeting one patient adopting a warm and open stance for one shift then increasing this to two more the next day.
R	**Realistic** goals will involve negotiation, and perhaps renegotiation with the student as to how they can develop the skill.
T	**Timely/time-based** – when will the student be able to demonstrate that they have developed effective communication skills, e.g. by the mid-point of their placement or nearer to the end?

5.9 WAYS TO ENCOURAGE STUDENTS TO ENGAGE WITH FEEDBACK

When feedback is turned into action it prompts a shift in student learning. When educators continuously link feedback to feedforward to role model the process then students will engage in that behaviour too (Day, 2019). Creating a toolkit for students to actively seek our feedback includes offering a list of questions. Edinburgh Napier University set up a student partnership project 'making connections with feedback' to co-create a tool for students to use in practice. It advocates that students require feedback literacy and suggests a number of questions that students can use to increase their understanding of and engagement with feedback:

- How do you think I am progressing? What do you think I am doing well? How could I improve further on that?
- What are the areas of my practice that you think need most improvement? Am I working at the right level?
- In the (named area) in which I am less confident, how could you help me improve?
- Where else could I gain support so I can keep improving?
- If you were in my shoes, how would you change your practice?
- Have I done (named practical task) well? What do you think?
- Is there a time when we can take 10 minutes and talk somewhere privately? If not, when would be the best time to talk?

- To help me deal with the feedback I receive, can you tell me how you yourself interpret and respond to feedback?
- I have a specific interest in (named specialism). What in your opinion would be the best steps to proceed in that direction?
- Where can I find research evidence or other information to help me expand my knowledge and make improvements in my practice?

It also offers advice on gaining the best possible feedback from your mentors and the following statements are based on Edinburgh Napier Student Partnership Project:

- Be proactive in seeking feedback: the more you ask, the more you are likely to receive
- Value the opinions of your practice supervisor, even if you disagree with them; listen carefully and respectfully; even if you interpret their words as harsh, you can still learn from them
- Question your own thoughts and actions out loud to your practice supervisor and ask for feedback on your ideas
- If feedback is given to you in passing, ask for clarification about anything you do not understand; explore both positive and negative feedback.

Table 5.5 is also based upon the Edinburgh Napier Student Partnership Project. This project between staff and students co-created this advice on how to manage common reactions to negative feedback and how to cope with it.

Table 5.5: *Edinburgh Napier Student Partnership Project*

Common emotional reactions to feedback	Ways to manage emotional responses
• Becoming defensive and arguing • Crying or feeling emotional • Being in denial, refusing to believe the comments or ignoring them • Taking the comments personally and assuming that you are at fault • Feeling as though there is nothing you can do about it • Dwelling excessively on negative feedback and allowing feedback to affect your progress or mental health • Failing to ask for feedback due to negative experiences	• Start by acknowledging to yourself how bad you feel • Sometimes you need time to reflect before feeling able to work with feedback • Ask questions to clarify what the particular problem is • Avoid (if possible) being excessively emotional in your responses – but don't be afraid to have a good cry in private • Seek advice and support from peers • Think about your supervisor – it may have been a bad day and not really all about you • Make sure that you continue to seek feedback so you can learn how to improve

5.10 MANAGING DIFFICULT CONVERSATIONS

Throughout your professional life you will need to engage in difficult conversations. If you avoid having difficult conversations, then the same issues will arise time and time again. If you have a staff member who constantly calls a student nurse 'the student', instead of using their name, then unless that individual has their behaviour pointed out to them as unacceptable, they may be completely unaware and think that this is acceptable. There will also be times when you are educating students in practice when you will have to speak to students about issues that might be personal and you know that it is going to be difficult for you, them or both of you.

 ACTIVITY 5.4

In order to start developing your confidence in tackling difficult conversations it can be useful to think back to previous difficult conversations that you have had and consider the following:

Question	Answer
Why have you found some conversations difficult?	
Have you avoided conversations that you thought would be challenging?	
What stopped you from holding these conversations?	
Are there any themes emerging?	
How can you develop from what you have learned from reflecting on these points?	

This is a personal reflective activity, so no answer guide is provided.

The prospect of having a difficult conversation can make us feel uncomfortable. There are a number of barriers which make conversations difficult:

- A power imbalance: you may fear that you could be construed as bullying a student by raising any concerns
- You have tried to sort the issue out with this person before and it has not worked
- You have left things alone to see if they improve without interference and now fear you have left it too long to address the issue
- You may not know how to go about resolving the issue
- There may be too many issues to confront
- There may be cultural barriers to resolving the issue
- You may feel intimidated by the person you need to speak to.

These barriers are not insurmountable and, in reality, professionals need to learn to deal with a variety of situations for which they feel initially underprepared. Having difficult conversations is inescapable, so therefore it is an area that nurses need to develop. If you are going to have to have difficult conversations then you may as well be well prepared for them. This is particularly important when you are involved in the development of the future of nursing, i.e. your role when you are educating student nurses.

In your practice area there may be a minor issue; for example, two members of your team have said to you that the student you are supervising is overfamiliar with patients, calling them pet names such as 'Grandad' or other names that they have not asked to be called. You understand that the student is shy and may be overcompensating in trying to establish a rapport with patients. You also understand that it is your duty to "act as an advocate for the vulnerable, challenging poor practice and discriminatory attitudes and behaviour relating to their care" (NMC, 2018c, p. 7) and also use your knowledge and skills for the benefits of people in your care and colleagues and to do this you must "provide honest, accurate and constructive feedback to colleagues" (NMC, 2018c, p. 10).

It may be helpful to consider adapting some of the key concepts from the theories surrounding breaking bad news. While these difficult conversations about personal performance or learning are not on the same scale or as significant as breaking bad news, there are some similarities where the techniques could be applied. Using the principles may help to give structure when having a difficult conversation. Utilising some of Buckman's (1992) principles may help you as a practitioner to scaffold onto your existing knowledge. Here the acronym PATIENT (*Table 5.6*) is used, so when you think about difficult conversations you can think of putting the patient or person first, even if the person is the learner.

Table 5.6: Difficult conversations: PATIENT

P	Prepare yourself: know as much as you can about the issue before you address it; ask the staff who reported it how many times it happened; what have they said or done to address the issue with the student?
A	Ask the student to meet with you for a discussion and name the issue you want to address; this action would fire a warning shot using terms from Buckman's (1992) guidance; in this case you would say: "I would like to meet with you to discuss using patients' preferred names"; plan a time when you may be less busy (if possible) so you can both talk
T	Think about respecting the student's privacy when you plan where to meet to discuss the issue; role model respect
I	Involve the student in the discussion and allow space for them to respond; expect an emotional response to this feedback; feedback often triggers emotional responses
E	Explain professional requirements and the use of people's preferred names; share your skills and experience to inform the student's practice
N	Negotiate an action plan with the student; explain how they can become involved in their own development and suggest ways they can inform their own practice (such as suggested reading); together you could use the SMART framework to create the action plan
T	Timetable in another meeting with the student to discuss their progress surrounding the issue

5.11 SUMMARY

This chapter has discussed the principles of good feedback for you to use as part of your educational toolkit in practice. It has defined feedback in order to enable you to consider ways to encourage students to become more engaged in their own development through proactively seeking out feedback. The chapter explored the concepts of power and empowerment and ways to work with students as partners. It offered a framework for practice supervisors to be able to create action plans in partnership with students and also guided you on effective ways to initiate peer-to-peer feedback in your placement areas. Lastly it considered ways you can become more skilled in having difficult conversations with student nurses in order to facilitate their development.

RECOMMENDED FURTHER READING

Adamson, E., King, L., Foy, L. *et al.* (2018) Feedback in clinical practice: Enhancing the students' experience through action research. *Nurse Education in Practice*, **31**: 48–53. doi: 10.1016/j.nepr.2018.04.012

REFERENCES

Brookhart, S.M. (2017) *How to give effective feedback to your students.* ASCD.

Buckman, R. (1992) *How to break bad news: A guide for health care professionals.* Johns Hopkins University.

Day, T. (2019) *Turning feedback into feedforward.* Macmillan. Available at: www.macmillanihe.com/blog/post/feedback-feedforward-trevor-day/ (accessed 14 August).

Dweck, C.S. (2011) *Mindset: Changing the way you think to fulfil your potential.* Little, Brown.

Francis, R. (2013) *Report of the Mid-Staffordshire NHS Foundation Trust Public Inquiry Executive Summary.* The Stationery Office.

Healey, M., Flint, A. and Harrington, K. (2014) *Engagement through partnership: students as partners in learning and teaching in higher education.* Higher Education Academy.

Hounsell, D. (2004) *Reinventing feedback for the contemporary Scottish university.* Paper presented at Quality Enhancement Workshop on *Improving feedback to students*, University of Glasgow, June 2004.

Mortiboys, A. (2012) *Teaching with emotional intelligence.* Routledge.

Murphy, P. and Morley, C. (2020) Feedback. In: Ghisoni, M. and Murphy, P. (editors) *Study skills: for nursing, health and social care.* Lantern.

Nicol, D.J. (2010) From monologue to dialogue: improving written feedback processes in mass education. *Journal of Assessment and Evaluation in Higher Education*, 35(5): 501–17.

Nicol, D.J. and Macfarlane-Dick, D. (2006) Formative assessment and self-regulated learning: a model and seven principles of good feedback. *Studies in Higher Education,* 31(2): 199–218.

Nursing and Midwifery Council (2018a) *Realising professionalism: Part 1: Standards framework for nursing and midwifery education.* NMC. Available at: www.nmc.org.uk/globalassets/sitedocuments/education-standards/education-framework.pdf (accessed 13 August 2020).

Nursing and Midwifery Council (2018b) *Realising professionalism: Part 2: Standards for student supervision and assessment.* NMC. Available at: www.nmc.org.uk/globalassets/sitedocuments/education-standards/student-supervision-assessment.pdf (accessed 13 August 2020).

Nursing and Midwifery Council (2018c) *The Code: Professional standards of practice and behaviour for nurses, midwives and nursing associates*. NMC. Available at: www.nmc.org.uk/globalassets/sitedocuments/nmc-publications/nmc-code.pdf (accessed 14 August 2020).

Race, P. (2014) *Making learning happen*. 3rd edition. Sage.

Sambell, K., McDowell, L. and Montgomery, C. (2016) *Assessment for learning in higher education*. Routledge.

Scott, K. (2017) *Radical candor: How to be a great boss without losing your humanity*. Macmillan.

Wilson, A. (2019) *Teaching intelligence: how to improve feedback conversations*. Times Higher Education. Available at: www.timeshighereducation.com/news/teaching-intelligence-how-improve-feedback-conversations (accessed 28 September 2020).

Winstone, N., Nash, R.A., Parker, M. and Rowntree, J. (2017) Supporting learners' agentic engagement with feedback: A systematic review and a taxonomy of recipience processes. *Educational Psychology*, **52**(1): 17–37.

ACTIVITY ANSWER GUIDE

ACTIVITY 5.1

Potential answers to the reflective questions:

1. Each shift; weekly; monthly; annually.
2. A lot of people would like more feedback than they receive. It may be worth considering how to motivate others to offer feedback on specific areas within your role to help you to maintain your own professional development.
3. Patients/peers/managers/students/other members of the team.
4. See *Section 5.9, Ways to encourage students to engage with feedback*: there is a list of questions that are aimed at students asking for feedback but could be developed for use by any healthcare professional.
5. The way you cope with feedback may have a bearing on how you give it to others. It is normal to have an emotional reaction (good or bad) to feedback. What is important is how you learn from it and how you can role model that learning to others.
6. This question presents you with an opportunity to ask each student how they want their feedback and negotiate ways that are beneficial to

both of you. In general feedback is best given as soon after the event as possible for it to have maximum effect. It needs to be offered in the spirit of growth and development and to enable the other party to learn from it.

7. Are you only offered feedback when you have done well/made a mistake/had a complaint made against you or the department? If you are not receiving balanced feedback then could you take ownership of this and start to ask for more regular feedback? Could the team offer peer support in this area?

CHAPTER 6

SUPPORTING STUDENTS THROUGH CHALLENGING PRACTICE SUPERVISION AND ASSESSMENT SITUATIONS

Elaine Beaumont, Gail Norris
and Caroline J. Hollins Martin

6.1 INTRODUCTION

This chapter explores strategies to cultivate compassion for self and others in the workforce. You will be introduced to self-soothing exercises designed to help you when making those difficult practice supervision and practice assessment decisions. This chapter also introduces the compassionate mind approach that when used by supervisors and assessors may help students experience a 'safe base' in which they can build resilience and an environment in which supportive conversations can take place. This chapter applies a scenario about Sarah, a student midwife who has experienced a challenging practice-based situation.

The emphasis within this chapter is on the midwifery scenario; however, it is important to realise that both nursing and midwifery students are likely to experience challenging situations. The chapter is written so that practice supervisors and practice assessors from both professional disciplines can adapt and apply these techniques with students in a range of contexts.

After reading this chapter you will be able to:
* Discuss the role of the Nursing and Midwifery Council (NMC) in providing standards that guide education of midwives
* Begin to use compassionate mind training
* Explore methods of cultivating compassion
* Use soothing exercises that create affiliative feelings for oneself and others.

To create the first paving slab of understanding, it is first important to define the role of a midwife.

6.1.1 Role of the midwife

The fact that human babies are born in each and every country across the world makes midwifery a truly global profession. Within the UK, midwives are fully accountable as the lead professional for the care and support of women, newborn infants, partners and families (NMC, 2019b). Midwives provide care based upon the best possible evidence and work in care providing partnership with women and their families. Midwives nurture normal physiological processes and support safe physical, psychological, social, cultural and spiritual practice. Midwives also aim to promote positive outcomes and to prevent complications developing (NMC, 2019b). Globally a midwife is a person who has successfully completed an educational programme that is based upon the International Confederation of Midwives (ICM) *Essential competencies for midwifery practice*, and the *Framework of the ICM Global Standards for Midwifery Education*. A midwife is an individual who has acquired the requisite qualifications to be registered to practice midwifery and use the title 'midwife' (NMC, 2019b).

6.1.2 The role of the NMC in providing standards that guide education of midwives

The NMC in the UK is the independent regulator for nurses, midwives and nursing associates. The NMC sets the standards for the professions it registers and is tasked with the responsibility of ensuring that the standards it sets remain contemporary and fit for purpose.

To ensure this, in 2016 the NMC launched its programme of change for midwifery education, during which it executed a major review of all its education standards. In response to the findings, the NMC published new standards that directed practice from 2018 onwards. As such, the nurses and midwives on the NMC professional register were consulted, alongside the wider health, social care and education communities across the four UK countries. The views of patients, carers and members of the public were sought for the purpose of determining necessary roles and proficiencies of the future midwife and nurse and the education programmes and practice learning experiences needed to prepare them for practice. The end-product was publication of the *Realising professionalism: Standards for education and training* (NMC, 2018a, b; 2019a) which consists of:

Part 1 Standards framework for nursing and midwifery education

These standards are set by the NMC to manage the quality of pre-registration nursing and midwifery programmes and post-registration programmes offered by approved academic educational institutions in partnership with practice learning partners (NMC, 2018a).

Part 2 Standards for student supervision and assessment

These standards are defined NMC expectations for learning, support and supervision of students in the practice environment (NMC, 2018b).

Part 3 Standards for pre-registration midwifery programmes

These standards are specified for each pre-registration programme. They set out legal requirements and include: entry requirements and entry routes, length of programme, curriculum, practice learning, supervision and assessment, and the qualifications to be awarded for all pre-registration midwifery programmes (NMC, 2019a). This standard for midwifery students stipulates that full training must be a minimum of 3 years and 46000 hours, or where a student is already an NMC registrant, full-time education shall be a minimum of 2 years and 3600 hours. The curricula must provide an equal balance of 50% theory and 50% clinical practice.

The above three standards must be used in conjunction with *Standards of proficiency for midwives* (NMC, 2019b) which apply to all NMC midwives. These standards are proficiencies that state outcomes that each midwife must achieve at the point of registration. The proficiencies are grouped under six domains that are interrelated and build upon each other:

- **Domain 1** Being an accountable, autonomous professional midwife
- **Domain 2** Safe and effective midwifery care, promoting and providing continuity of care and carer
- **Domain 3** Universal care for all women and newborn infants
- **Domain 4** Additional care for women and newborn infants with complications
- **Domain 5** Promoting excellence: the midwife as colleague, scholar and leader
- **Domain 6** The midwife as a skilled practitioner.

Several key themes run throughout the domains, including evidence-based care; the importance of staying up-to-date; the physical, psychological, social, cultural and spiritual safety of women; communication and relationship building with women; advocating for the human rights of women and children; and working across the whole continuum of care and in all settings (NMC, 2019b).

6.1.3 The role of education institutions

Education institutions must comply with all NMC standards if they want to run any NMC-approved programmes. Approved educational institutions, together with practice learning partners, must comply with the whole of the NMC standards set.

6.2 STUDENT SUPPORT IN THE LEARNING ENVIRONMENT

The implementation of the NMC (2018b) *Part 2: Standards for student supervision and assessment* provides each student with a practice supervisor, practice assessor and academic assessor; these roles have been discussed in detail in *Chapter 2*. It may be useful to refer to the roles when continuing to read and work through this chapter.

6.2.1 A practice scenario that could arouse challenging emotions

For you the reader to understand the necessity of equipping students with strategies to build resilience and cultivate self-compassion, a scenario (*Scenario 6.1*) will now be described that is likely to arouse challenging feelings and emotions in the student's mind. Remember that while this scenario is specific to midwifery, there are times when practice encounters are difficult and challenging for both student nurses and midwives.

 SCENARIO 6.1

Sarah is a second-year student midwife, currently working with her practice supervisor in the birthing centre.

Sarah was caring for Anna and her partner, and this was Anna's second baby. Anna's first birth had resulted in a shoulder dystocia. Her last baby weighed 4kg. Anna continued to labour very quickly and soon felt the urge to push. Sarah, although mindful of Anna's past obstetric history, was confident as she had just completed a session in the simulation centre in university, where she was able to practise the manoeuvres that practitioners can use to deal with this extremely difficult situation. As Anna approached the second stage of labour, Sarah was able to encourage Anna to adopt an all-fours position to give birth. Anna's labour progressed quickly, and she began to push. The vertex became visible very quickly; however, the baby's face and chin delivered very slowly. The 'turtle sign', where the head recoils against the perineum was evidence that this was again another shoulder dystocia. Sarah pressed the emergency buzzer and, with guidance from her practice supervisor, quickly supported Anna to move onto her back and assume McRobert's position with

SCENARIO 6.1 *(cont'd)*

suprapubic pressure applied. The obstetric emergency team quickly arrived and proceeded to use internal manoeuvres to attempt to manipulate the baby to rotate into an oblique position and under the symphysis pubis. Eight minutes later, a male baby was born with an Apgar 2 at 1 minute. Resuscitation was immediately performed. Following an unsuccessful attempt to resuscitate, Anna's baby boy was pronounced dead.

Immediately following this incident, Sarah was encouraged by her practice supervisor to reflect on this event using a reflective model. The thought of returning to the delivery suite the following day filled Sarah with fear and anxiety. Sarah phoned in sick to her clinical placement and didn't return for 3 days. Two weeks on, Sarah is still finding it difficult to accept the death of Anna's baby, because they had followed a structured framework to deal with this obstetric emergency and the baby still died. How can this be?

Sarah recounted numerous times, over and over again in her head, the events that led to the death of Anna's baby. Had she done anything wrong? Were the parents blaming her? Were her peers thinking she'd made a mistake? She is now feeling anxious, has self-critical thoughts and wants to leave her midwifery training behind. To help Sarah reflect and work her way through this event, her practice supervisor, practice assessor and academic assessor have all agreed to meet.

6.2.2 Explaining the scenario

Should dystocia occur when either the anterior, or less commonly, the posterior fetal shoulder impacts upon the maternal symphysis pubis, it is termed an obstetric emergency, since there is an elevated risk of a 'shoulder dystocia' ending in fetal death or maternal morbidity or mortality (Stables and Rankin, 2010). A shoulder dystocia can be an unpredictable event, but it does require urgent manoeuvres to attempt to manipulate the fetal shoulder into an oblique plane in the maternal pelvis and under the maternal symphysis pubis (Stables and Rankin, 2010). Maternal morbidity is increased, particularly in the event of a postpartum haemorrhage (risk = 11%). In addition, third- and fourth-degree perineal tears may occur (risk = 3.8%) (Royal College of Obstetricians and Gynaecologists (RCOG), 2012). Complications for the baby include: birth asphyxia, meconium aspiration and brachial plexus injury, with the latter most common (risk = 2.3–16%) (RCOG, 2012; Stables and Rankin, 2010).

There is an expectation that student midwives, upon qualification, can demonstrate the necessary skills to respond to obstetric emergencies. However, the reality is that they are rare events (Norris, 2008), with the incidence of shoulder dystocia being between 0.58 and 0.70% of births (RCOG, 2012). These figures create a challenge for midwifery educators, who are responsible for ensuring that student midwives are fit for practice (Norris, 2008). In clinical practice, in the event of an obstetric emergency, the midwife often assumes the leadership role and the student midwife becomes the observer. This in itself leads to questioning how the student midwife learns the appropriate skills to manage an obstetric emergency.

 TOP TIP

While this chapter looks specifically at an emergency situation that takes place in a midwifery setting, there are many situations in clinical practice that are unpredictable and where the outcomes are not always positive. Unpredictable emergency situations can arise at any time, in any clinical setting. Do therefore read and use the content of the chapter in relation to your supervisory and assessment role.

 SCENARIO

In relation to the comment made by Sarah in the scenario:
The thought of returning to the delivery suite the following day filled Sarah with fear and anxiety. In response, she phoned in sick and did not attend her clinical placement for the subsequent 3 days.

The Davies and Coldridge (2015) study, which explored traumatic experiences of student midwives in clinical practice, highlights that while the focus at the beginning of midwifery programmes is upon normal birth, many students in this study reported experiencing traumatic births early in their clinical experience. Some of the participating students cited stress as a factor in their decision to leave the programme.

Sarah's emotional response to this traumatic event is not uncommon. Davies and Coldridge (2015) describe the emotional response of other students who have witnessed traumatic events in clinical practice, with descriptions of overwhelming responsibility they experienced during an emergency event. These students described emotional responses to traumatic events that included withdrawal, low mood, fearfulness, emotional distress and guilt. Some students were unable to allay fears about their own competence and, like Sarah in the scenario, described that they worried about whether they could or should have helped more. Some of these students expressed worry in relation to their levels of resilience in the face of events, along with fear of potential long-term consequences and litigation. These feelings are not unique to UK student midwives, with 15% of Swedish obstetricians and midwives reporting symptoms of partial or probable post-traumatic stress disorder (PTSD) post experiencing severe traumatic events in the 'birthing unit' (Wahlberg *et al.*, 2016).

Hunter and Warren (2014) emphasise the nature of close working one-on-one midwife-to-woman relationships, which can place midwives at potential risk of suffering emotional stress, especially when problems arise during childbirth. The word midwife means 'with woman', which involves midwives being involved in highly empathetic relationships with clients. During pregnancy and labour, the evolving close relationship between woman, partner and family has potential to increase stress experienced by the midwife, particularly when care has been invested and a subsequent trauma occurs (Showalter, 2010).

Hunter and Warren (2014) recognise that workplace pressures and the emotional demands of the job may increase midwives' experience of stress and contribute to low morale, sickness and programme attrition. Hence, there is a need to build resilience within the midwifery workforce. Resilience is a word that describes relative resistance to adversity (Rutter, 1999). The term includes the ability of an individual to draw on effective resources and respond positively and consistently to adversity, through implementation of effective coping strategies (Seery *et al.*, 2010). This responsive need to build resilience in student midwives within curriculum has been acknowledged by the NMC (2019b). In response, strategies to build student resilience must now be included within UK midwifery curriculum. Garrosa *et al.* (2010) recognise that certain factors can mediate resilience, which includes positive perceptual and attributional styles, self-actualisation, self-awareness, reflexivity, self-efficacy and using active coping strategies.

Students' personal awareness can be developed through self-reflection (Grafton *et al.*, 2010), which is a well-used tool embedded as a method of teaching, learning and assessment within UK midwifery curriculum (NMC, 2019a). Nonetheless, Hunter and Warren (2014) emphasise the need for educators to implement additional methods of building resilience, with additional support required when students experience a traumatic event in clinical practice. Using self-reflection as an educational tool for professional development is important, simply because it enables discovery, uncovering and analysing knowledge to evidence-based clinical practice (Lyons, 1999).

In the stated scenario, Sarah's practice supervisor telephoned her and arranged a meeting with her, which required both her practice assessor and her academic assessor to be present. Sarah was encouraged by her practice supervisor to self-reflect upon this incident, through use of a reflective model. Self-awareness, description, critical analysis, synthesis and evaluation are the cognitive and affective tools required to engage in reflection (Atkins and Murphy, 1993). Hence, by encouraging Sarah to actively reflect upon her thoughts, feelings and emotions, this process actively encourages the development of effective coping mechanisms.

Lyons (1999) recognises that encouraging students to reflect upon their experience fosters a spirit of inquiry and improves knowledge and ability to develop skills of critical analysis. Experience plays an important role in the learning process and provides practical knowledge that can inform professional action (Lyons, 1999).

 SCENARIO

In relation to Sarah's scenario:
To help Sarah navigate her way through her traumatic practice-based event, her practice supervisor, practice assessor and academic assessor have all agreed to meet with Sarah.

The study by Seibold (2005) explored a cohort of Bachelor of Midwifery student midwives' experiences of mentorship/preceptorship and found that the most helpful mentors/preceptors were those that provided a debrief following a critical incident or traumatic event. Analysis of such trauma-arousing events can trigger negative and positive emotional responses, which can be discussed during a debrief session.

6.3 HOW DOES CLINICAL SUPERVISION WORK IN THE CONTEXT OF STUDENT TRAUMA?

Clinical supervision in the context of *Scenario 6.1* is applied whereby the practice supervisor, practice assessor and academic assessor have all agreed to meet with Sarah to provide the support.

Supervision in a trauma-focused context should include a restorative component, which encourages students to find resolution through an exploration of the scenario (Raab, 2014). Processes involve examining aspects that have touched the student emotionally, with emphasis placed upon improving capacity and reducing symptoms associated with traumatic stress and burnout that stem from emotional, psychological, physical and spiritual exhaustion (Klimecki and Singer, 2012). Responding to one's own suffering with compassion can have a positive impact on the student midwife and enhance their education (Beaumont and Hollins Martin, 2016; Key *et al.*, 2019). This approach encourages students to reflect upon their trauma event within a safe space, with learning gained designed to reduce related stress (Bishop, 2007; Wallbank, 2010). This restorative component is designed to help equip the student midwife with reflective skills that may help them better manage taxing clinical work (Sheen *et al.*, 2014). In this context, supervision involves reflecting upon events and examining what went well or otherwise and how improvements can be made in developing a positive and quality relationship between supervisor(s) and student.

There are a variety of tools that can be applied to practice supervision and used to aid analysis of the chosen clinical scenario such as the one presented so far in this chapter that focuses on Sarah, with a collaborative and trusting relationship essential for supervision to be effective.

Three elements can help build resilience: (1) *Respond*, (2) *Reflect* and (3) *Restore* (Key *et al.*, 2019).

The goal is to build resilience through *Reflecting* upon the trauma event and how the student *Responded* and why. During this process attempts are made to *Restore* emotions to a comfortable position. Post *Responding* and during the process of *Reflecting*, the *Restore* component involves the supervisor(s) placing emphasis upon processing emotions and building the student's resilience to cope in a similar future event.

The rationale for reflecting upon traumatic experiences is because experience alone does not lead to insightful learning (Loughran, 2002). Ordinarily, students like Sarah are not straightforwardly reflecting upon the event, but are also required to focus consciously on emotions, experiences and responses in attempts to reach an elevated position of understanding (Paterson and Chapman, 2013). It is important to understand that, due to our preferred ways of thinking and responding, we all have a propensity to repetitively engage in self-limiting behaviours (Turesky and Gallagher, 2011). Challenge can be helpful towards breaking the cycle (Helsing *et al.*, 2008). Reflection that is performed well has the ability to shift anxiety into positive energy and address the gap between actual and desirable practice. There are many reflective models available to analyse a traumatic event.

For example, Gibbs' reflection cycle (1988) provides a circle of steps to guide the process (see *Figure 6.1*):

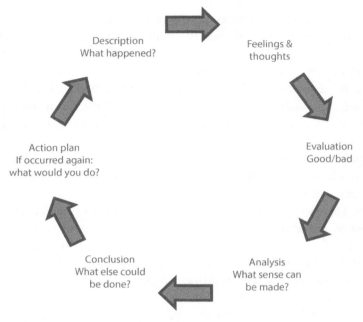

Figure 6.1: *Gibbs' reflective model (adapted from Gibbs, 1988).*

Relating back to *Scenario 6.1* with Sarah, during the process of reflecting upon the woman's traumatic event, it is important that the practice supervisor, practice assessor and academic assessor provide affirmations for the student, which can comprise assertions, support, verification, confirmation and encouragement. Such affirmations can help the students like Sarah learn to cope with threat and its associated stress, and by doing so act towards improving their confidence to work in the clinical area. At the end of the session, it is important to assess the student's views of the reflection session, e.g. what has gone well and what has not. In addition, techniques that aim to reduce threat-based thinking and emotions can aid student development.

☰ TOP TIP

As a practice supervisor, practice assessor or academic assessor, you might want to rehearse these conversations with your team or with peers, before having them with learners.

6.4 COMPASSIONATE MIND TRAINING

Introducing students, whether they are midwives or nursing students, to interventions that promote self-compassion is useful, simply because it teaches strategies that aim to bring balance to emotional upset. According to Klimecki and Singer (2012), compassion fatigue can potentially be averted through exercises that activate neural pathways associated with compassion, empathetic concern, positive feelings and altruistic behaviour.

Gilbert (2005, p. 217) defines compassion as a quality that: "aims to nurture, look after, teach, guide, mentor, soothe, protect, offer feelings of acceptance and belonging". Compassionate mind training (CMT) is designed to enhance levels of compassion, help bring balance to emotional systems and reduce self-criticism (Beaumont and Hollins Martin, 2015; Raab, 2014). Beaumont *et al.* (2016) examined relationships between wellbeing, self-compassion, compassion for others, compassion fatigue and burnout in student midwives (*n* = 103). Just over half of the sample reported above average scores for burnout. The results indicate that student midwives who report higher scores on the self-judgement subscale are less compassionate towards both themselves and others, have reduced wellbeing, and report greater burnout and compassion fatigue. Student midwives who report high on measures of self-compassion and wellbeing report less compassion fatigue and burnout.

6.4.1 Why a CMT approach?

A compassion-based approach is appropriate because there is a growing body of neuroscientific evidence that has demonstrated that motives and emotions have a major impact upon self and affect regulation (Depue and Morrone-Strupinsky, 2005). CMT aims to help the person respond to self-criticism and threat-based emotions with compassion, with the goal to improve psychological wellbeing. A key part of the process is to help the student understand that many cognitive biases and distortions are built-in biological processes constructed by genetics and the environment (Gilbert, 2014).

Compassion-focused therapy (CFT) was founded by Professor Paul Gilbert (2000) in response to the observation that many people, in particular those populations high in shame and self-criticism, experienced difficulties generating kind and self-supportive inner voices when participating in traditional therapeutic approaches such as cognitive behavioural therapy (CBT). Gilbert observed that although these individuals were able to engage with cognitive and behavioural tasks, they often responded poorly to therapy (Bulmarsh *et al.*, 2009; Rector *et al.*, 2000). Also, systematic and narrative reviews about CFT have shown it to be effective as an intervention in reducing symptoms of trauma and complex post-traumatic stress disorder (CPTSD) in other populations (Beaumont and Hollins Martin, 2015; Karatzias *et al.*, 2019; Leaviss and Uttley, 2015). There are several models of compassion, all of which show a negative relationship between compassion and psychopathology (MacBeth and Gumley, 2012).

The MacBeth and Gumley (2012) meta-analysis reports a large effect size for relationships between compassion and depression and anxiety and stress, with high levels of compassion associated with lower levels of psychopathology. Several studies have explored relationships between self-compassion and wellbeing. For example, survey research using scales of self-compassion shows that self-compassion correlates with wellbeing (Neely *et al.*, 2009; Neff *et al.*, 2007).

An increase in levels of self-compassion also correlates with a decrease in psychiatric symptoms, interpersonal problems, personality pathology (Schanche *et al.*, 2011) and psychological wellbeing (Van Dam *et al.*, 2011).

In response to this evidence, Beaumont *et al.* (2016) concluded that midwifery students could benefit from learning to be 'kinder to self' when faced with challenging circumstances. Hence, cultivating environments that foster compassion can help student midwives cope with clinical, organisational and educational demands (Beaumont, 2016). There is no reason why this could not extend and apply to nursing students. As such, developing interventions that cultivate compassion will improve students' ability to cope with distress by reducing levels of self-critical judgement and self-attack. The act of self-compassion involves responding to self-suffering with a non-judgemental attitude, kindness and understanding (Neff *et al.*, 2007). According to Neff (2003) there are three elements of self-compassion: (1) *self-kindness*, (2) *common humanity* and (3) *mindfulness*. Self-kindness is linked with patience and understanding of oneself, and common humanity recognises that all people make mistakes. In response, mindfulness takes a non-judgemental view when the student midwife experiences negative emotions.

6.4.2 *Bringing balance to the threat, drive and soothing systems*

Gilbert (2000, 2009) suggests that we have three systems that have evolved over millions of years to protect us, drive us forward and to help us rest, soothe and recuperate. Let's take a closer look at each one in turn.

Threat and protection system

This system alerts us and directs our attention to things that we experience as threatening and dangerous. The emotions we feel when this system is online include anger, anxiety and disgust, all of which prompt the body into action. This system creates 'better safe than sorry' scenarios that focus on the negative. When the threat system is triggered, we tend to imagine worst-case scenarios, get caught up in rumination and thinking–feeling loops.

Individuals who have high levels of self-criticism or shame tend to have a dominant threat system (Beaumont and Hollins Martin, 2016; Gilbert, 2009, 2010). For example, a midwife engaged in an unexplained stillbirth may worry they will be shamed, blame themselves for the outcome, or ruminate about what their supervisors and peers may think about their part in the scenario. It may be worth thinking about analogous nursing student practice learning situations that may lead to high levels of self-criticism such as the unsuccessful resuscitation of a patient.

Drive system

This system motivates us to pay attention to resources that will be potentially helpful – it's our doing, wanting and achieving system. When activated we experience emotions such as excitement and joy, which reinforce behaviour. Status-seeking, competitiveness and working to avoid rejection are also associated with this system (Depue and Morrone-Strupinsky, 2005).

Soothing/affiliative system

This system is associated with physiological responses including calming, soothing, attachment and interpersonal connection (Depue and Morrone-Strupinsky, 2005; Gilbert, 2014). We can learn to cultivate behaviours that soothe and reduce the symptoms linked with the threat system by cultivating compassion, feelings of safeness and social connection. When we receive compassion from others this creates 'in-group' security and can help us regulate the three systems. Cultivating this system involves helping individuals to learn to care for their wellbeing and become more mindful of their own and other people's needs (Gilbert, 2014).

6.4.3 How the systems interact

CMT aims to bring balance by building the soothing affiliative system, understand how the three systems impact upon one another and bring compassion to self-criticism.

Compassion as a flow

Compassion flows in three ways (Gilbert, 2014):
1. Compassion for others (*compassion flowing out*)
2. Compassion from others (*compassion flowing in*)
3. Self-compassion (*self-to-self compassion*).

Teaching CMT

Experiencing clinical trauma can take its toll, with CMT potentially building emotional resilience through making the student feel 'cared for' by self and others. CMT consists of cultivating the soothing system by using:
• Breathing exercises that focus on slowing the body down
• Imagery and memory to calm and soothe the mind
• Method-acting techniques (experiencing what it would be like to be a compassionate self)
• Recalling experiences of both giving (to self and others) and receiving compassion
• The skills of compassionate attention and mindfulness, compassionate engagement with emotion, compassionate thinking and compassionate behaviour.

Compassionate letter writing, and bringing compassion to shame and self-criticism, fears and blocks are also important components.

Measuring effects

There are several scales that can be used to measure before and after effects of a CMT intervention. For example:
• Compassionate engagement and action scales (Gilbert *et al.*, 2017)
• The forms of self-criticising/attacking scale (FSCRS) (22 items) (Gilbert *et al.*, 2004)
• Self-compassion scale (Neff, 2003)
• Professional quality of life scale (Stamm, 2009)
• Short Warwick and Edinburgh mental wellbeing scale (Tennant *et al.*, 2009).

CMT implementation for student midwives

A full teaching programme of CMT can be accessed in a paper written by Beaumont and Hollins Martin (2016). While written for student midwives, the programme also applies to student nurses. During the process student midwives and nurses:

- Are introduced to core elements of Gilbert's (2009) model
- Explore the evolved nature of the human mind
- Review how a sense of self is created by genetics and social experience
- Learn how shame and self-criticism impact upon levels of compassion
- Carry out experiential exercises designed to cultivate distinct aspects of compassion.

In summary, CMT aims to balance the threat, drive and soothing systems, which can be achieved by utilising the attributes and skills of compassion. Within the context of supervisors and *Scenario 6.1* involving Sarah, the student midwife, Gilbert (2009) would advise that the supervisor develop their:

- Awareness of Sarah's suffering
- Turn towards Sarah's suffering
- Have ability to tolerate and engage with Sarah's distress, as opposed to avoiding, denying or dissociating from her suffering
- Help Sarah cultivate compassion for her own suffering.

A second and further aspect of compassion involves the supervisor acknowledging and knowing what to do when suffering is experienced (Gilbert, 2014). Compassionate attributes (the first psychology of compassion) and compassionate skills (the second psychology of compassion) are of key importance (see *Table 6.1*).

Table 6.1: Outline of the skills and attributes in providing compassion

Compassionate attributes – engaging with distress	Compassionate skills
Care for wellbeing: Developing a caring motivation and wish to alleviate and turn toward suffering	*Attention*: Focusing our minds on things that are helpful and not harmful; paying attention in the moment – in the here and now
Sensitivity to distress: Recognising and being attentive to one's own and other people's distress	*Imagery*: Using imagery to create feelings of calm and to stimulate the soothing systems
Sympathy: The ability to be emotionally moved by feelings of distress rather than feeling disconnected from it	*Sensory*: Using breathing practices, vocal tones, facial expressions and body postures to generate physical states and to help regulate distress
Distress tolerance: Being able to tolerate difficult emotions by moving toward suffering rather than avoiding suffering	*Reasoning*: Learning to reason in ways that are helpful, compassionate and caring
Empathy: Being in tune emotionally with somebody who is suffering	*Feeling*: Learning to compassionately respond to emotions
Non-judgement: The process involves stepping back from judgement, self-criticism and condemnation	*Behaviour*: Behaving in ways that are helpful for self and others; this can sometimes take courage

Creating conditions in which midwives and nurses feel safe, valued, accepted and cared for, may work towards reducing threat-based fear (Beaumont, 2016). Helping people engage with their own suffering also fosters compassionate caregiving and provides a secure base (Bowlby, 1969) to practitioners.

Using Sarah in *Scenario 6.1* as an example, Sarah is doubting herself, has symptoms of anxiety (palpitations and rumination), has critical thoughts, is worried about returning to work, thinks she is not good enough and has started to worry about what her peers think of her. Let us look at some interventions that practice supervisors, practice assessors and academic assessors may apply to help Sarah cultivate compassion for her own suffering and traumatic experience. The idea is that everyone can engage in these activities; but as a practice supervisor, practice assessor or academic assessor you might want to teach students how to use these techniques.

6.4.4 Attention

Explaining that 'what we focus on expands' could help Sarah. Our attention can be directed, it can be moved. Strengthening 'our attention muscles' can lead to a variety of benefits for both physical and mental health (Irons and Beaumont, 2017). When we train our attention, we start to notice when our mind wanders. We can gently and kindly return it to things that are less stressful, and we can use our breath, sound and our body as an anchor for our mind (Irons and Beaumont, 2017).

Sarah's attention is caught up in rumination and she has started to worry about what people think of her. To distract Sarah's attention, she can learn to switch her focus.

It is recommended that you try *Activity 6.1* so that you have experienced sound as an anchor for attention.

✎ ACTIVITY 6.1

Mindfulness of sound
  Follow the instructions in *Box 6.1* and then answer the reflective questions:
1. How did it feel to use sound as an anchor for your mind and attention? If you noticed your mind wandered, were you able to bring your attention back to the sounds around you?
2. How could you use this activity with Sarah or for one of your students?

This is a personal reflective activity, so no answer guide is provided.

Box 6.1: *Mindfulness of sound*

Find a comfortable place to sit, adopting an upright posture. For 30 seconds or so, just become aware of your body sitting in the chair, and for a moment or so, your breath as it moves in and out of your body. When you feel ready, see if you can slowly allow your attention to broaden away from your body. Start to become aware of the sounds that you can hear around you. To start with, try not to reach out to the sounds, but rather be receptive as they arise and disappear around you. Let them come to you – you are in this moment, just paying attention to the sound as it arises. Become aware of the direction they arise in, and their nature – what their character is, volume, tone, pitch or whether they are constant or intermittent. Try to notice when your mind has become distracted – this might be by thoughts or concerns that pop into your mind or emotional reactions to the sounds – and once aware, try, to the best of your ability, bringing your mind back to noticing the sounds around you again.

For 60 seconds or so, see if you can focus your attention more purposefully on one sound that you can hear around you. Really try to use this as an anchor for your attention. Notice with curiosity the nature and characteristics of this and return to this sound if your mind wanders. After a while try to pull back from focusing on this sound and see if you can split your attention and notice or become aware of all of the sounds you can hear around you, so that no sound is paid more attention to than others. Repeat this process, focusing on just one sound for a period, and then pulling the focus back to become aware of all sounds.

When you're ready, widen your awareness to the room around you … bring yourself to the present moment.

From Irons and Beaumont (2017) *The compassionate mind workbook: A step-by-step guide to cultivating your compassionate self*, reprinted with kind permission from Little, Brown.

6.4.5 Soothing rhythm breathing

The way we breathe can have a powerful impact on our body. Actors, singers, sportsmen and sportswomen are taught to breathe in ways that help them deliver their best performance. The way we breathe influences our nervous system, triggers feelings, behaviour and specific thinking patterns. Activating the parasympathetic nervous system by creating a soothing rhythm breathing (SRB) pattern could help Sarah regulate heart rate and slow her mind and body down, giving herself time to rest and recuperate.

It is recommended that you participate in *Activity 6.2*, learning how to slow your breathing.

ACTIVITY 6.2

Learning to slow down – how to slow your breathing
Follow the instructions in *Box 6.2* and then answer the following reflective questions:
1. What was your experience of engaging a soothing breathing rhythm?
2. What did you notice about your thoughts, physical sensations and feelings?
3. What future stressful situations could be helped by doing this exercise?
4. Did you experience any difficulties doing the exercise? For example, did you find yourself distracted by thoughts or sensations? If so, try not to judge or criticise yourself; with practice you will find the exercise easier.

This is a personal reflective activity, so no answer guide is provided.

Box 6.2: *Learning to slow down – how to slow your breathing*

Find a quiet and comfortable place to sit. Take a moment to embody the grounded, upright, confident posture you have practised in *Activity 6.1*. If you feel comfortable, close your eyes. If not, rest your gaze directly ahead of yourself, with your head in an alert, upright position. Begin by bringing your attention to your breathing in a mindful way. Notice the sensations present as you breathe in and out. If you notice that your attention becomes distracted, and moves away from your breath, just observe this and gently try to bring your attention back to your breath, without judging or criticising yourself that this has happened.

Now, as you are gently holding your attention in the flow of your breath, gently try and bring a soothing or calming rhythm breathing to your body. This is likely to be a slower and deeper rhythm than usual, but one that feels comfortable and natural to your body. Try if you can to breathe in a smooth, even way. If you notice your attention moving away from your breath, or that you become distracted in any way, gently bring your attention back to your breath and tune back in to the calming or soothing quality of your breathing rhythm.

Now, see if you can slow your breathing down a little further. Sometimes it can be worth counting your breath to start with. For example, try breathing in to the count of five, with each count representing a second. Once you've got to five, hold for one second before breathing out for five seconds (again counting to five as you do so). Hold for the count of one, before breathing in again to the count of five.

Out-breath 1 – 2 – 3 – 4 – 5

Hold 1

In-breath 1 – 2 – 3 – 4 – 5

Hold 1

Out-breath 1 – 2 – 3 – 4 – 5

Hold 1

In-breath 1 – 2 – 3 – 4 – 5

Continue – roughly in this rhythm – for another 2 or 3 minutes, staying connected with your soothing rhythm breathing. When you are ready, widen your awareness to the room around you … notice the sounds in the room and bring yourself to the present moment.

From Irons and Beaumont (2017) *The compassionate mind workbook: A step-by-step guide to cultivating your compassionate self*, reprinted with kind permission from Little, Brown.

 TOP TIP

The aim of SRB is to engage the soothing system to help us be alongside difficult experiences when they arrive. So, practising when we are OK can help us prepare for when we face tricky, stressful or difficult situations. Repeating phrases such as 'mind slowing down' and 'body slowing down' could also help you find a steady, calm breathing rhythm (Irons and Beaumont, 2017).

6.4.6 *Imagery*

Creating a calm, peaceful place using guided-imagery interventions aims to cultivate the soothing system. It is recommended that you participate in

Activity 6.3, creating an image of a place in your mind that makes you feel safe, calm and soothed.

☑ ACTIVITY 6.3

Follow the instructions in *Box 6.3* and then answer the following reflective questions:

1. What was it like to create an image of a calm, special, soothing place for yourself?
2. What could you see and smell? What physical sensations did you notice?
3. What was it like to be welcomed by this place you created in your 'mind's eye'?

This is a personal reflective account, so no answer guide is provided.

Box 6.3: Creating an image of my safe place

Find somewhere comfortable to sit where you will not be disturbed. Take a few moments to adopt your grounded, upright, confident body posture. Engage in your soothing rhythm breathing, allowing your breathing and body to slow down a little.

When you feel ready, spend some time bringing to mind an image of a place that you feel is safe, soothing or calming in some way. This may be somewhere you have been before or somewhere completely 'made up'. Try not to get frustrated or worried if no image comes to mind for a while, or if you find that several different images come to mind. Mindfully try and stay with the intention to allow an image to come to mind that feels safe, calming or soothing in some way.

When an image has come to mind, spend a few moments being with it. To start with, mindfully pay attention to what you can see in this image. This might be colours, shapes or objects. Spend 30 seconds doing this. Next, notice if there are any sounds that are present in this image or your safe place. If there are, gently pay attention to these, noticing the different qualities they may have, how they leave you feeling. Spend 30 seconds or so doing this. Now, notice whether there are any soothing or comforting smells that are present here in your image. If there are, again spend 30 seconds paying attention to this. Next, notice any physical sensations you can feel or things you come into physical contact with or touch, such as the warmth of the sun against your skin or the feel of the grass, or sand beneath your feet. Focus on this for 30 seconds. Maybe you can consider whether you are in your safe place on your own, or whether someone or something else (like an animal) is there with you.

As this is your own safe place, imagine that it has an awareness of you. It welcomes you there, and is happy to see you; it wants you to feel safe and calm. Notice how it feels to know that this place wants you to feel supported, safe and at ease. Spend a minute or so just focusing on this.

Given that this is a place in which you can feel at ease, calm and safe, it may be useful to consider what you would like to do while being here. Maybe you wish to remain still, content with just 'being' in the moment, in this place. Or you might like to explore the place in a more active way, or moving around in this place, walking, swimming or playing a game. It is your own unique safe place, you can use it in a way that helps you to feel at ease, as well as engaged and interested, with the freedom to explore.

When you're ready, widen your awareness to the room around you … notice the sounds in the room and bring yourself to the present moment.

From Irons and Beaumont (2017) *The compassionate mind workbook: A step-by-step guide to cultivating your compassionate self*, reprinted with kind permission from Little, Brown.

6.4.7 Thinking

Sarah is worrying about returning to work, ruminating about what her peers and supervisors think of her, and consequently she has feelings of doubt and self-criticism. To help alleviate these thoughts, Sarah can develop self-compassion to address her critical self, which has the purpose of developing more balanced thinking. One method of addressing this is to generate supportive and compassionate statements, which can help Sarah move away from rumination and self-criticism. Some examples follow, which demonstrate empathy for distress, compassionate attention, compassionate thinking and compassionate behaviour:

- Life can be hard. Other people have also experienced situations like this and they also have found it hard.
- I have managed troubles in the past. Think about what helped me in these previous situations.
- It is understandable that I feel like this. This event was shocking and sad, and it is difficult to experience another person suffering.
- I am starting to notice when my threat system is activated. When it is activated, I am likely to have biased 'all or nothing' thoughts.
- There are people who care about me and want to help me through this experience.
- I have thousands of thoughts every day, and need to remember that many thoughts are not facts.
- Speaking to friends at work and family about how I am feeling, will help me come to terms with this situation.
- These feelings will pass.

Sarah could also be encouraged to think about what she would say to a friend who was in a similar situation. We tend to be kinder and more compassionate to others, compared with what we show to ourselves.

6.4.8 Emotion

Identifying our emotions is beneficial to wellbeing. Examining our emotions can help us figure out:

1. What happens in our body when we experience intense emotions (heart rate may change, voice reverberate and/or feeling like we want to vomit)
2. How often we experience a labelled emotion (e.g. Sarah may notice that she is experiencing anxiety more than sadness or fear)
3. What happens to thinking patterns when we experience difficult emotions (e.g. Sarah's thoughts may include: "I can't cope", "what do others think?", and/or "I cannot do this any longer")

4. What the emotion is driving us to do (e.g. in Sarah's case, anxiety may cause her to have thoughts about hiding away whereas, and in contrast, fear might guide her to avoid future scenarios, and as such abandon her profession).

☑ ACTIVITY 6.4

Consider the following:
   If Sarah imagines a friend or colleague in the same scenario, she may begin to think and feel in a more balanced way. If Sarah imagines listening to narratives of anxiety, low mood, fear and shock spoken by someone she cares about, she may start to experience the situation differently. What would she say to a friend or colleague if the roles were reversed?
   This is a personal reflective account, so no answer guide is provided.

When a person experiences threat, there are tendencies to use strategies (e.g. run away, overeat, use alcohol, etc.) that drown out difficult and responsive emotions. When such a situation arises, it is important for the person to express what they feel. Hence, it could be helpful for you to ask them the following:

- Imagine you are at your compassionate best. How might your compassionate self help you express how you feel?
- Would it help to talk to somebody else about how you feel?
- Would it help to write down how you feel?
- Would it help to ask a friend, colleague or family member for support?
- Would it help to practise talking about how you feel out loud, possibly while looking in the mirror?
- How can you show compassion to the part of you that is struggling?
- If you struggle with expressing how you feel, would it help to observe how other people express their emotions? (e.g. consider the voice tone, body language and facial expression of others). Could you practise using a similar tone, expression and body language when you offer compassion and care to yourself?

6.4.9 Behaviour

Creating a pre, during and after (PDA) plan (not to be confused with public displays of affection) could help Sarah's nervousness about returning to placement.

Professional sportswomen and sportsmen prepare for an event, game or match by creating a plan. For example, footballers prepare for matches by taking penalties repeatedly, and tennis players practise serves and winning shots before a match. Pre the event, athletes eat certain foods, create a practical plan in their mind, exercise, do warm-ups and stretches, imagine scoring the winning goal or visualise themselves on a podium being awarded the gold medal. Similarly, Sarah can carry out relaxation exercises, use soothing rhythm breathing, and provide supportive inner self-talk. For example, 'you got this' or 'you can do this'. With similarity to the athlete, post-event Sarah can do warm-downs and review her performance with her supervisor (coach).

Before returning to her placement, Sarah should be encouraged to practise SRB, imagine her calm soothing place and create a list of supportive statements. This plan can be written down in an action plan developed with her supervisor. On the first day of return, Sarah could spend a portion of time conducting breathing exercises, repeating her supportive statements, holding an object that reminds her to show compassion and kindness to self, and remind herself that her internal thoughts are not facts. After the return day, Sarah can take a balanced review of her day, and make sure she reflects upon what went well. Also, Sarah can be encouraged to write a reflective compassionate letter to herself, in which she addresses what she has learned from the scenario and in which she praises herself for facing her anxieties. A PDA template (Irons and Beaumont, 2017) can be used to help plan for other difficult situations (see *Table 6.2*).

Table 6.2: A pre, during and after (PDA) plan

Difficult situation	Pre	During	After

6.5 SUMMARY

This chapter has explored strategies that aim to cultivate compassion for self and others in the workforce. You have been introduced to some of the practices and skills used in CMT and, through the activities you have experienced, how the exercises and reflections can cultivate the soothing system and help practice supervisors and practice assessors support themselves and their students. Developing assessors and supervisors who understand the compassionate mind approach may help students experience a 'safe base' in which supportive and challenging conversations can take place.

RECOMMENDED FURTHER READING

Beaumont, E., Durkin, M., Hollins Martin, C.J. and Carson, J. (2016) Compassion for others, self-compassion, quality of life and mental well-being measures and their association with compassion fatigue and burnout in student midwives: A quantitative survey. *Midwifery*, **34**: 239–44. doi.org/10.1016/j.midw.2015.11.002

Beaumont, E. and Hollins Martin, C.J. (2016) Heightening levels of compassion towards self and others through use of compassionate mind training. *British Journal of Midwifery*, **24(11)**: 3–12. doi. org/10.12968/bjom.2016.24.11.777

Gilbert, P. (2009) *The compassionate mind*. Constable.

Irons, C. and Beaumont, E. (2017) *The compassionate mind workbook: A step-by-step guide to developing your compassionate self*. Little, Brown.

REFERENCES

Atkins, S. and Murphy, K. (1993) Reflection: a review of literature. *Journal of Advanced Nursing*, **18**: 1188–92.

Beaumont, E. (2016) A compassionate mind training model for healthcare practitioners and educators. *Healthcare Counselling and Psychotherapy Journal*, **16(3)**: 22–7.

Beaumont, E., Durkin, M., Hollins Martin, C.J. and Carson, J. (2016) Compassion for others, self-compassion, quality of life and mental well-being measures and their association with compassion fatigue and burnout in student midwives: A quantitative survey. *Midwifery*, **34**: 239–44.

Beaumont, E. and Hollins Martin, C.J. (2015) A narrative review exploring the effectiveness of compassion-focused therapy. *Counselling Psychology Review*, **30(1)**: 21–32.

Beaumont, E. and Hollins Martin, C.J. (2016) Heightening levels of compassion towards self and others through use of compassionate mind training. *British Journal of Midwifery*, **24(11)**: 3–12.

Bishop, V. (2007) *Clinical supervision in practice*. 2nd edition. Palgrave Macmillan.

Bowlby, J. (1969) *Attachment: Attachment and loss*. Volume 1. Hogarth.

Bulmarsh, E., Harkness, K.L., Stewart, J.G. and Bagby, R.M. (2009) Personality, stressful life events, and treatment response in major depression. *Journal of Consulting and Clinical Psychology*, **77**: 1067–77.

Davies, S. and Coldridge, L. (2015) No man's land: An exploration of the traumatic experiences of student midwives in practice. *Midwifery*, **31**: 858–64.

Depue, R.A. and Morrone-Strupinsky, J.V. (2005) A neurobehavioral model of affiliative bonding: implications for conceptualizing a human trait of affiliation. *Behavioral and Brain Sciences*, **28**: 313–49.

Garrosa, E., Rainbo, C., Moreno-Jimenez, B. and Monterio, M. (2010) The relationship between job stressors, hardy personality, coping resources and burnout in a sample of nurses: a correlational study at two time points. *International Journal Nursing Studies*, **47**: 205–15.

Gibbs, G. (1988) *Learning by doing: a guide to teaching and learning methods*. Further Education Unit.

Gilbert, P. (2000) The relationship of shame, social anxiety and depression: The role of the evaluation of social rank. *Clinical Psychology and Psychotherapy*, **7**: 174–89.

Gilbert, P. (2005) Social mentalities: A biopsychosocial and evolutionary reflection on social relationships. In: Baldwin, M. (editor) *Interpersonal cognition*. Guilford.

Gilbert, P. (2009) *The compassionate mind*. Constable.

Gilbert, P. (2010) *Compassion focused therapy: The CBT distinctive features series*. Routledge.

Gilbert, P. (2014) The origins and nature of compassion focused therapy. *British Journal of Clinical Psychology*, **53(1)**: 6–41.

Gilbert, P., Catarino, F., Duarte, C. *et al.* (2017) The development of compassionate engagement and action scales for self and others. *Journal of Compassionate Health Care*, **4(1)**: 4.

Gilbert, P., Clark, M., Hempel, S., Miles, J.N.V. and Irons, C. (2004) Criticising and reassuring oneself: An exploration of forms, styles and reasons in female students. *British Journal of Clinical Psychology*, **43**: 31–50.

Grafton, E., Gillespie, B.M. and Henderson, S. (2010) Resilience: the power within. *Oncology Nurse Forum*, **37**: 698–705.

Helsing, D., Howell, A., Kegan, R. and Lahey, L.L. (2008) Putting the "development" in professional developing: understanding and overturning educational leaders' immunities to change. *Harvard Educational Review*, **78(3)**: 437–65.

Hunter, B. and Warren, B. (2014) Midwives' experiences of workplace resilience. *Midwifery*, **30**: 926–34.

Irons, C. and Beaumont, E. (2017) *The compassionate mind workbook: A step-by-step guide to cultivating your compassionate self*. Little, Brown.

Karatzias, T., Murphy, P., Cloitre, M. *et al.* (2019) Psychological interventions for ICD-11 complex PTSD symptoms: systematic review and meta-analysis. *Psychological Medicine*, **49(11)**: 1761–75.

Key, S., Marshall, H. and Hollins Martin, C.J. (2019) The Scottish clinical supervision model for midwives. *British Journal of Midwifery*, **27(10)**: 655–63.

Klimecki, O. and Singer, T. (2012) Empathic distress fatigue rather than compassion fatigue? Integrating findings from empathy research in psychology and social neuroscience. In: Oakley, B., Knafo, A., Madhaven, G. and Wilson, D.S. (editors) *Pathological altruism*. Oxford University Press.

Leaviss, J. and Uttley, L. (2015) Psychotherapeutic benefits of compassion-focused therapy: an early systematic review. *Psychological Medicine*, **45**: 927–45.

Loughran, J. (2002) Effective reflective practice: in search of meaning in learning about teaching. *Journal of Teacher Education*, **53(1)**: 33–43.

Lyons, J. (1999) Reflective education for professional practice: discovering knowledge from experience. *Nurse Education Today*, **19**: 29–34.

MacBeth, A. and Gumley, A. (2012) Exploring compassion: a meta-analysis of the association between self-compassion and psychopathology. *Clinical Psychology Review*, **32**: 545–52.

Neely, M.E., Schallert, D.L., Mohammed, S.S., Roberts, R.M. and Chen, Y.J. (2009) Self-kindness when facing stress: The role of self-compassion, goal regulation, and support in college students' well-being. *Motivation and Emotion*, **33(1)**: 88–97.

Neff, K.D. (2003) The development and validation of a scale to measure self-compassion. *Self and Identity*, **2**: 223–50.

Neff, K.D., Kirkpatrick, K.L. and Rude, S.S. (2007) Self-compassion and adaptive psychological functioning. *Journal of Research in Personality*, **41**: 139–54.

Norris, G. (2008) The midwifery curriculum: Introducing obstetric emergency simulation. *British Journal of Midwifery*, **16(4)**: 232–5.

Nursing and Midwifery Council (2018a) *Realising professionalism: Part 1: Standards framework for nursing and midwifery education*. NMC. Available at: www.nmc.org.uk/globalassets/sitedocuments/education-standards/education-framework.pdf (accessed 13 August 2020).

Nursing and Midwifery Council (2018b) *Realising professionalism: Part 2: Standards for student supervision and assessment*. NMC. Available at: www.nmc.org.uk/globalassets/sitedocuments/education-standards/student-supervision-assessment.pdf (accessed 13 August 2020).

Nursing and Midwifery Council (2019a) *Realising professionalism: Part 3: Standards for pre-registration midwifery programmes*. NMC. Available at: www.nmc.org.uk/globalassets/sitedocuments/standards/standards-for-pre-registration-midwifery-programmes.pdf (accessed 17 August 2020).

Nursing and Midwifery Council (2019b) *Standards of proficiency for midwives*. NMC. Available at: www.nmc.org.uk/globalassets/sitedocuments/standards/standards-of-proficiency-for-midwives.pdf (accessed 17 August 2020)

Paterson, C. and Chapman, J. (2013) Enhancing skills of critical reflection to evidence learning in professional practice. *Physical Therapy in Sport*, **14**(3): 133–8.

Raab, K. (2014) Mindfulness, self-compassion, and empathy among health care professionals: a review of the literature. *Journal of Health Care Chaplaincy*, **20**(3): 95–108.

Rector, N.A., Bagby, R.M., Segal, Z.V., Joffe, R.T. and Levitt, A. (2000) Self-criticism and dependency in depressed patients treated with cognitive therapy or pharmacotherapy. *Cognitive Therapy and Research*, **24**: 571–84. doi.org/10.1023/A:1005566112869

Royal College of Obstetricians and Gynaecologists (2012) *Green top guideline no. 42: shoulder dystocia*. Royal College of Obstetricians and Gynaecologists.

Rutter, M. (1999) Resilience concepts and findings: Implications for family therapy. *Journal of Family Therapy*, **21**(2): 119–44.

Schanche, E., Stiles, T.C., McCullough, L., Svartberg, M. and Nielsen, G.H. (2011) The relationship between activating affects, inhibitory affects, and self-compassion in patients with Cluster C personality disorders. *Psychotherapy*, **48**: 293–303.

Seery, M.D., Holman, E.A. and Silver, R.C. (2010) Whatever does not kill us: cumulative lifetime adversity, vulnerability and resilience. *Journal of Personality and Social Psychology*, **99**: 1025–41.

Seibold, C. (2005) The experiences of the first cohort of Bachelor of Midwifery students. *Australian Midwifery Journal*, **18**: 9–16.

Sheen, K., Slade, P. and Spiby, H. (2014) An integrative review of the impact of indirect trauma exposure in health professionals and potential issues of salience for midwives. *Journal of Advanced Nursing*, **70**: 729–43.

Showalter, S.E. (2010) Compassion fatigue: What is it? Why does it matter? Recognizing the symptoms, acknowledging the impact, developing the tools to prevent compassion fatigue, and strengthen the professional already suffering from the effects. *American Journal of Hospice and Palliative Care*, **27**: 239–42.

Stables, D. and Rankin, J. (2010) *Physiology in childbearing: with anatomy and related biosciences.* 3rd edition. Baillière Tindall.

Stamm, B.H. (2009) Professional quality of lifescale: Compassion satisfaction and compassion fatigue version 5 (ProQOL). Available at: https://proqol.org/ProQol_Test.html (accessed 17 August 2020).

Tennant, R., Hiller, L., Fishwick, R. *et al.* (2009) The Warwick and Edinburgh mental well-being scale (WEMWBS): Development and UK validation. *Health and Quality of Life Outcomes*, **5(63)**: 1–13.

Turesky, E.F. and Gallagher, D. (2011) Know thyself: coaching for leadership using Kolb's experiential learning theory. *The Coaching Psychologist*, **7(1)**: 5–14.

Van Dam, N.T., Sheppard, S.C., Forsyth, J.P. and Earleywine, M. (2011) Self-compassion is a better predictor than mindfulness of symptom severity and quality of life in mixed anxiety and depression. *Journal of Anxiety Disorders*, **25**: 123–30.

Wahlberg, A., Andreen Sachs, M., Johannesson, K. *et al.* (2016) Post-traumatic stress symptoms in Swedish obstetricians and midwives after severe obstetric events: a cross-sectional retrospective survey. *BJOG An International Journal of Obstetrics and Gynaecology*, **124(8)**: 1264–71. doi:10.1111/1471-0528.14259

Wallbank, S. (2010) Effectiveness of individual clinical supervision for midwives and doctors in stress reduction: findings from a pilot study. *Evidence Based Midwifery*, **8**: 65–70.

CHAPTER 7

WHAT IS ASSESSMENT AND WHAT ARE WE ASSESSING?

Debbie Roberts

7.1 INTRODUCTION

In previous work I have explored the concept of assessing student nurses' clinical learning. According to Roberts (2011, p. 607):

> *"the drift towards competency-based nurse interventions has seen a growth in concern regarding the most appropriate methods of assessment of such competencies. Nurse educators and practitioners alike are struggling with the concept of measuring the performance of nursing skills; due to an uneasy relationship between competence, capability, intuition and expertise. Different currencies of value may be ascribed to the assessment of nursing practice, resulting in the use of subjective judgements together with the development of assessment criteria which have different weightings, depending on the values of the assessor".*

The new Nursing and Midwifery Council (NMC) standards for student supervision and assessment (NMC, 2018c) outline new roles of practice supervisor and practice assessor to support student learning in and through clinical practice. The standards of proficiency for registered nurses (NMC, 2018a) describe specific outcome statements and proficiencies that students must achieve in order to join the NMC register. These outcomes and proficiencies must be demonstrated when caring for people of all ages across a wide range of clinical settings. Under the new standards the NMC makes clear that student assessment must be:

> *"evidence based, robust and objective. Assessments and confirmation of proficiency ... based on an understanding of student achievements across theory and practice".* (NMC, 2018c, p. 8)

Practice assessors are therefore required to conduct objective, evidence-based assessments of students, providing constructive feedback to facilitate professional development in others, and demonstrating knowledge of the assessment process and their role within it (Leigh and Roberts, 2018).

This chapter provides an overview of the nature of clinical assessment and explores what it means to be proficient. The skills of assessment are outlined together with some exercises to encourage readers to develop their questioning and assessment skills. The chapter discusses how practice assessors will cope with students on different programmes at varying academic levels; for example, students that already have a degree in and may be undertaking a master's level pre-registration nursing programme. A range of approaches to assessment are discussed and linked to the NMC requirement for practice assessors to link with academic assessors. The role of patients or service users in assessment will also be discussed.

After reading this chapter you will be able to:
- Discuss the role of the practice assessor
- Identify a range of individuals where you work that practice assessors should link with
- Identify and apply criteria that you (and other assessors where you work) have agreed and will use to measure student performance against the NMC standards.

7.2 THE PRACTICE ASSESSOR

The **practice assessor** is one of three new roles developed by the NMC as part of the 2018 *Future nurse: Standards of proficiency for registered nurses* (NMC, 2018a). The practice assessor must be a nurse (while other allied professionals can participate formally in student support and learning, they should not undertake summative assessment of student nurses) and should assess students' understanding in relation to theory and practice. There is also a mandate that under normal circumstances individuals cannot act as both supervisor and assessor to the same students, but may occupy these new roles for different students.

The practice assessor:
- Conducts assessments to confirm the student's achievement of proficiencies and programme outcomes for practice learning
- Makes assessment decisions that are informed by feedback sought and received from practice supervisors

- Makes and records objective, evidence-based assessments on conduct, proficiency and achievement, drawing on student records, direct observations, student self-reflection and other resources
- Works in partnership with the nominated academic assessor to evaluate and recommend the student for progression for each part of the programme, in line with programme standards, and local and national policies
- Should have sufficient opportunities to observe the student periodically across environments in order to inform decisions for assessment and progression (NMC, 2018c).

Practice-based assessment should therefore be informed by feedback from a range of professionals (other practice supervisors) and should be detailed, robust and thorough. Practice assessors are expected to: "... undertake preparation or evidence prior learning and experience that enables them to demonstrate achievement of minimum outcomes" (NMC, 2018c). There is an expectation that supervisors and assessors will be provided with ongoing support and training, and will be able to reflect on, and develop in, the role. Individuals are required to continue to develop their professional practice and knowledge proactively to fulfil their role. Furthermore, ongoing development will be achieved in different more contemporary ways compared with the previous standards; for example, through attendance at conferences, engaging in simulation, and use of coaching skills, action learning and distance learning.

ACTIVITY 7.1

If you have been asked to take on the role of practice assessor, how do you plan to uphold these requirements? What support mechanisms might you require?

This is a personal reflective activity, so no answer guide is provided.

As a practice assessor, you will be required to assess the student's ability to make connections between various pieces of information and theory and make links to the clinical situation at hand. In other words, you will be assessing both theoretical and practical knowledge. The *Future nurse: Standards of proficiency for registered nurses* (NMC, 2018a, p. 3), refer to: "knowledge and skills registered nurses must demonstrate when caring for people of all ages and across all care settings". The knowledge proficiencies that are expected of registrants are grouped under seven platforms and are accompanied by two annexe documents containing nursing procedures.

7.3 ASSESSMENT PRACTICES

Providing honest and consistent judgements about students' performance in clinical practice has long been a requirement in nurse education in the UK. Assessments which take place in the fast-paced environment of clinical practice can be fraught with difficulty. According to Cassidy:

> *"competence should be concerned with the ability to master specific clinical skills and possess necessary personal characteristics to function effectively as a nurse including the capacity for reflection. In addition, however, competence assessment also needs to be balanced with the student's ability to apply technical prowess and personal attributes to the local context of care situations".* (Cassidy, 2009, p. 34)

The NMC is concerned with proficiency and all nurses, regardless of the academic level at which they study, are deemed to have the same level of proficiency at the point of registration.

ACTIVITY 7.2

Before moving on, let us consider one of the NMC (2018a) outcome statements in relation to assessment and what it is that an assessor might value:
Outcome statement 3.14 (p. 15):

> *"Identify and assess the needs of people and families for care at the end of life, including requirements for palliative care and decision-making related to their treatment and care preferences".*

What might you expect a student nurse to demonstrate against this outcome statement?

Now imagine how the context of nursing practice might influence your thoughts; for example if you work in a unit that cares for people with dementia, as opposed to working in mental health with people with low mood, how might this influence what you would expect the student to demonstrate?

You might also want to think about the impact of end of life across the age continuum; for example, if a child is at the end of life would you expect the student to demonstrate different knowledge and skills? Should different knowledge and skills be demonstrated according to the context of care?

You might feel that students would not have an opportunity to learn or be assessed against this particular outcome statement; if so, look at one of the other outcome statements under Platform 3: *Assessing needs and planning care*, and think about the questions posed here.

An answer guide is provided at the end of the chapter.

Following a narrative review of 23 global papers, Helminen *et al.* (2016) confirm previous ideas about the lack of consistency of assessing students in clinical practice. The subjective bias of assessors remains an area of concern. Within the findings of the review, Helminen *et al.* (2016) describe how competency and competence assessment are variously interpreted. In the assessment of clinical practice, it remains unclear what exactly is being given value. The relationship between competence, confidence, knowledge, expertise and skills is an uneasy one (Roberts, 2011).

The questions posed here might make you think of a range of knowledge and skills that you would expect the student to demonstrate; these are effectively the criteria that you will use to make a judgement about whether the student is proficient in this area of practice. However, these word-based criteria pose a problem in terms of assessment: assessors in clinical practice may not all be looking for the same thing. Word-based criteria are open to interpretation and there may be a lack of agreement between different assessors as to what is meant by these criteria. This can result in the criteria being interpreted differently by different people in the same clinical setting or between different clinical settings, all of which can be very confusing for the student.

ACTIVITY 7.3

There may be a number of practice assessors in the area where you work. It might be useful to try and have a group discussion to try and reach a consensus as to what things you will be looking for against a range of outcome statements, so that you can try to minimise differences in your approach and improve the consistency of your assessments.
An answer guide is provided at the end of this chapter.

Kajander-Unkuri *et al.* (2016, p. 305) precis three main approaches to conceptualising competence based on available literature:
- Behaviouristic – based on tasks and skills
- Generic – focused on transferable attributes, and
- Holistic – bringing together knowledge, skills, attributes and values.

The majority of literature agrees that competence is an amalgamation of knowledge, skills and attitudes (or behaviours) but: "what is not agreed is how each of these elements can be applied to make definitive assessments of competence" (Zasadny and Bull, 2015, p. 127). Indeed, even the terms knowledge, skills and attitudes are open to interpretation and debate.

Assessment of students in clinical practice is challenging for assessors; perhaps no more so than when a student's performance is marginal or borderline between pass or fail.

(Note: some higher education institutions and clinical placement providers will grade a student's clinical performance while others will use a binary pass/fail approach.)

In an Australian study of 23 assessors, Hughes *et al.* (2019) demonstrate that organisational processes significantly impacted on assessors; in particular, time demands and pressures, assessment processes and learning and teaching practices. While it should be remembered that the system of nurse education in Australia is different to that of the UK, there are still some important messages within this paper. The authors describe how university processes, such as whether or how a student can appeal a decision, influenced assessment decisions:

> "*Some assessors had positive experiences with the appeals process and felt that it was well structured, others found it to be a difficult process for all parties. The majority of participants discussed the need for ample evidence to support a recommendation to fail a student, which impacted on assessors' workload and feelings of being questioned and unsupported. Many assessors only put forward a fail recommendation if they felt they had strong evidence to withstand an exacting appeal, even if they knew the student did not meet professional standards*". (Hughes *et al.*, 2019, p. 246).

Hughes, Johnston and Mitchell go on to suggest that often workload pressure and time can mean that assessors might be inclined to pass a student, especially if the placement is relatively short; exacerbating the feeling of not having enough time to work with and formally assess students.

In a grounded theory study conducted in the UK, Cassidy *et al.* (2017) explored experiences of assessing nursing students on the borderline of achievement of competence in clinical practice. The study highlights the importance of the collaboration between assessors, other colleagues and higher education staff (and others). The nature of the relationships between these parties could authorise or disempower the assessor's decisions one way or another in borderline cases. The study reinforces the importance for teams to develop an assessor community where there is an agreement about what is being assessed and what is being looked for (the criteria) (Cassidy *et al.*, 2017).

7.4 TYPES OF ASSESSMENT

Opinions vary as to the number of different types of assessment. The Open University provides an excellent overview of the definition of assessment together with some learning resources related to different types of assessment:

www.open.edu/openlearn/ocw/mod/oucontent/view.php?id=20113& section=2

Here we will focus on formative and summative assessment and explore the way in which continuous and episodic assessment can be undertaken.

Formative assessment is useful because it enables the students to rehearse what will happen during the more formal summative assessment. As such, formative assessment is often viewed as an informal process where the learner is provided with feedback and support on their performance in order to learn. Formative assessment shifts the focus from assessment of learning to one of assessment for learning (Boud and Soler, 2016). The paper by Boud and Soler provides a useful overview of a range of what they refer to as sustainable assessment methods. Formative assessment relies on feedback; this is discussed more fully elsewhere in this book (see *Chapter 5*).

Formative feedback and reflection tools have been devised for use in high-fidelity simulation; for example, see Solheim *et al.* (2017) in *Recommended further reading.*

Summative assessment is a formal process where assignments are marked or graded. In practice learning terms, nursing practice is not always graded, but students' competence or proficiency is judged as either pass or fail.

Levett-Jones *et al.* (2011) describe the Structured Observation and Assessment of Practice (SOAP) model. This model could be described as episodic assessment because of the nature of the time frames where the student is assessed. SOAP is a practice-driven model of assessment taking place in clinical practice over the course of two 3-hour observation periods. During the course of the observation period, students are encouraged to engage in their usual patient care activity. There are several elements to the assessment process including observation of student practice, mapping of student competencies against the requirements of the in-country professional standards and a viva. This approach seems particularly useful in assessing pre-registration students in the period immediately prior to qualification, since their ideas should be well developed by this point in the programme.

For further information download the article by Levett-Jones *et al.* (2011) from *References.*

7.4.1 The ASAP model

The Amalgamated Students Assessment in Practice model is presented by Zasadny and Bull (2015); it is known by the acronym ASAP meaning 'as soon as possible', because the model functions as a personalised early intervention strategy. The model is suggested as a useful assessment tool, a clinical reasoning framework and a negotiated learning contract (Zasadny and Bull, 2015). The tool also incorporates two other criteria-based tools or frameworks, namely ASK (attitudes, skills and knowledge) and SEP (safe, effective and proficient) together with a clinical reasoning framework. The model forms the basis of a feedback template to provide learners with detailed information about their performance and progress. As such, the model is used both formatively and summatively as a focused early diagnostic tool, a tool to provide evidence regarding the reasons why a learner might be struggling or failing to achieve in clinical practice. It can also be used to support the removal of students from the practice arena (Zasadny and Bull, 2015).

Download the paper by Zasadny and Bull (2015); in particular, look at how the model is used to provide detailed feedback to a student; see the table on p. 131 of the paper, which shows how ASK and SEP are used within the model, and how students can be provided with a narrative to justify assessment decisions in relation to clinical reasoning. Initial evaluations of the model in use in practice are promising. You might want to think about whether this framework would be useful where you work to structure assessment feedback.

☑ ACTIVITY 7.4

Try to plan ways in which the model could be used to provide feedback against a range of NMC (2018a) *Future nurse: Standards of proficiency for registered nurses* standard outcome statements; consider how you would use the framework to:

- Give positive feedback and praise to a student that has managed a particular patient encounter well
- Highlight areas where performance should be improved, or where an aspect of practice did not meet the required standard.

This is a personal reflective activity, so no answer guide is provided.

7.4.2 Ways to assess

An integrative literature review of 18 papers by Forber *et al.* (2016) highlights three main approaches to supervision in clinical practice:
- The traditional model whereby a clinical facilitator acts as primary instructor for a group of students
- The preceptorship model, essentially a 1:1 supervisory relationship between student and employed registered nurse
- Collaborative or partnership models, where all staff engage in student support.

The paper also outlines a range of other approaches including hub and spoke models and student wards. While not specifically about assessment methods, it is possible to draw conclusions regarding the manner of assessment associated with each of the approaches described by Forber *et al.* (2016).

Assessment can also be achieved by directly observing what the student does. For an outline of the impact of observation as a means of assessment in medical education, see LaDonna *et al.* (2017) in *Recommended further reading*.

ACTIVITY 7.5

Having read the paper describing medical education (LaDonna *et al.*, 2017), consider whether the impact of being observed would be similar for nursing students. Think about how as a practice supervisor you would observe students: would you tell students that you are observing their performance? And how would you know that the practice assessor will be looking for the same things?

This is a personal reflective activity, so no answer guide is provided.

For a comparable nursing paper, see Lamb and Norton (2018) in *Recommended further reading*.

Finally, assessment can be achieved by indirect or team assessment. This approach relies on good communication between individuals that work with the student. This regular communication about the students' progress will help to ensure that assessments are robust and evidence-based. Assessment can be undertaken by one individual or a team of people. It may involve close or direct observation or indirect observation. The NMC encourages local innovation and flexibility in how students are supervised and assessed. As a registrant, you may be engaged in different forms of supervision and assessment over the course of your career, or in different organisations. Try to ensure that you keep a reflective account to provide evidence of this activity as part of your revalidation requirements.

7.5 SELF-ASSESSMENT

Self-assessment is an important part of the assessment process and is suggested to stimulate deeper thinking and problem solving (Kajander-Unkuri *et al.*, 2016). Self-assessment is used in the UK and Australia (among others) to review feedback from patients and to enable students to consider competence and is seen as a skill associated with lifelong learning.

ACTIVITY 7.6

Download the paper by Kajander-Unkuri *et al.* (2016) from the reference list and read the section on p. 305 (paragraph 2) that describes various definitions of self-assessment in nursing.
- Think about whether you use any of the modes of self-assessment yourself as a practice supervisor or assessor.
- How might you use self-assessment as a tool when you are preparing to give students feedback on their performance?

This is a personal reflective activity, so no answer guide is provided.

Importantly, the study in Finland by Kajander-Unkuri *et al.* (2016) highlights that students may assess their own nursing competence more favourably than others, such as supervisors or assessors. The authors present some interesting discussion points regarding some of the potential reasons for the disparity (p. 309), such as differing understandings of competence, an overemphasis on skills-based nurse education and different reference points related to context or clinical area.

7.6 PATIENT/CLIENT/CONSUMER/SERVICE USER ENGAGEMENT IN ASSESSMENT

 TOP TIP

Note the different descriptive terms used here; you might want to think about the language used where you work.

For some time, authors have argued that service users should be actively engaged in all stages of professional education, including curriculum design, teaching delivery, assessment and evaluation (Warne and McAndrew, 2004). This movement is rooted in the belief that while academics (and others) may bring clinical or academic knowledge to the piece, only those who have experienced nursing care can bring a genuine voice of experience to bear. Indeed, Happell and Roper (2010) describe the title and role of consumer academic to cement the position of the voice of experience.

The NMC (2018b) *Part 1: Standards framework for nursing and midwifery education* contains five headings which higher education institutions must provide in order for a pre-registration programme to be validated by the professional governing body. You can access this part of the standards here: www.nmc.org.uk/globalassets/sitedocuments/education-standards/education-framework.pdf

There are several statements that relate to service user engagement generally and others which specifically relate to assessment:

> "*1.12 ensure programmes are designed, developed, delivered, evaluated and co-produced with service users and other stakeholders*" (p. 6)
>
> "*2.7 ensure that service users and representatives from relevant stakeholder groups are engaged in partnership in student recruitment and selection*" (p. 7)
>
> "*5.14 a range of people including service users contribute to student assessment*" (p. 12).

It is important to note here that decisions regarding summative assessment must be made by a nurse (for nursing students) or a midwife (for midwifery students), but that the NMC has recognised the importance of the contribution of others, such as service users, to the assessment process. The Health and Care Professions Council (HCPC) (2017, p. 32) also contains a standard requiring service users and carers to be involved in regulated programmes. Despite this requirement for service user engagement in assessment, examples within the literature are lacking. McSherry and Duggan (2016) provide one example related to carers being involved in the assessment of advanced practice master's level students (although it seems that these assessments were classroom based).

One example of service user involvement in practice-based feedback to mental health nursing students is described by Speers and Lathlean (2015): a feedback system was designed to enable students to "learn from rather than about service users" (p. 84).

☑ **ACTIVITY 7.7**

Read the paper by Speers and Lathlean (2015) from the reference list.
Reflect on your ideas about the relationship between professionals and service users. How do your ideas compare to those expressed in the paper? Think about whether this paper has challenged your ideas? In terms of implementing service user engagement in feedback or assessment where you work, could you start to think about ways in which this might be achieved?
This is a personal reflective activity, so no answer guide is provided.

The study by Speers and Lathlean (2015) refers to students asking for feedback from patients rather than patients engaging in the practice-based assessment of students, but nonetheless both students and service users appeared to benefit from the process. "An increased interchangeability between the helped and the helper" (Speers and Lathlean, 2015, p. 88) was evident.

7.7 ASSESSMENT AS AN EMOTIONAL ENDEAVOUR

It has long been known that supporting and managing a student who is struggling or failing in practice is an emotional endeavour (Duffy, 2003). Duffy's seminal work on failing to fail examined the factors that influence decisions surrounding the competence of nursing students. In later work, Duffy and Hardicar (2007) called for greater exploration of the emotional aspects of assessing student nurse competence, in particular a greater understanding of decisions regarding students who straddle the borderline between passing and failure, and for more research to explore student views of the system.

A study by Black *et al.* (2014) describes the experiences of nineteen mentors from seven healthcare organisations in South East England of failing an incompetent student in their final placement prior to qualifying. The study highlights that moral courage is key. Three themes are presented which together describe the moral courage required to fail a finalist student, these being:

> "*framed within the context of experiencing moral stress (the personal price), demonstrating moral integrity (professional responsibility and accountability) and ensuing moral residue (having the strength to fail final placement students but feeling powerless to do little to address a prevailing culture of failing to fail) with the overall synthesis being that these mentors' stories presented a new horizon of moral courage*". (Black *et al.*, 2014, p. 229).

Indeed, the data extracts presented by the authors are very powerful, and clearly portray the emotional aspects associated with failing a student. The participants describe being placed in a position of moral uncertainty because they had assumed that previous mentors should have addressed the students' shortcomings relating to fundamental areas of practice. Nonetheless, the mentors in the study all reached moral certainty in knowing that they were duty bound to fail such students in order to protect the public and uphold the integrity of the profession.

The strength of feeling expressed by the participants in Black *et al.* (2014) is even more interesting and pertinent when read alongside the findings from a later study by Hunt *et al.* (2016) who explored the coercive strategies used by students to try and exert influence over mentor/ sign-off mentor decisions. Hunt *et al.* (2016) point out that some of the behaviours described within the data may be 'unthinkable' to some within the profession; these behaviours described in the study are summarised in *Table 7.1*.

Table 7.1: Student behaviours (adapted from Hunt et al., *2016)*

Ingratiators	Aggressors
Students who curried favour with mentors by deliberate efforts such as being charming, obliging, indulging or emotionally exploitative; mentors were susceptible to high levels of guilt and low levels of fear when students employed these tactics Students often had likeable personalities and worked to sway mentors by doing things to please them such as bringing in cakes and making cups of tea, running errands, offering compliments or flattery or using persuasive emotional tactics like begging to be passed or overt demonstrations of emotions such as hugging or crying	Students engaged in open hostility towards mentors following negative feedback, threatening mentors verbally or physically both directly or indirectly through a third party; mentors experienced high levels of fear but minimal levels of guilt; mentors deeply affected by the lengths that students and their families would go to, e.g. threats touching their home life; student behaviour was so severe that it vindicated their decision to fail
Diverters	**Disparagers**
Students attempted to distract and redirect the mentor's focus: playing on factors unconnected to the areas of underperformance; incorporating elements such as illness, personal circumstances, disability or ongoing university proceedings; difficult for mentors to separate the relevant from the irrelevant and they were concerned that they might inadvertently be unreasonable; causing anxiety	Students who challenged their mentors in belittling, denigrating or professionally harmful ways, either by questioning the mentor's reasonableness and competence, or by accusations of harassment, bullying or discriminatory behaviour; guilt prompted the mentors to question themselves, increasing levels of fear as they envisioned ensuing investigation which might focus on their competence as a nurse, failings in supporting students or displaying prejudice or intimidation; they felt that students were not accustomed to frank critique

ACTIVITY 7.8

If there are a number of practice assessors where you work, try and have a group discussion about how such behaviours might be responded to or managed. In particular, you might want to consider what peer support you could provide each other in such circumstances. Read the suggestions put forward by Black *et al.* (2014) and discuss with your fellow practice assessors how you could implement these suggestions where you work.

This is a personal reflective activity, so no answer guide is provided.

The data presented by Hunt *et al.* (2016) and Black *et al.* (2014) are powerful. Importantly, Black *et al.* (2016) present mechanisms that could be considered to help (in this case) mentors in managing coercive students. Later work by Hunt (2019) describes some personal attributes and qualities of those individuals who would fail underperforming students; Hunt terms this as developing a 'core of steel', and identifies qualities: solidarity, tenacity, audacity, integrity and dependability. These are summarised in *Table 7.2* (Hunt, 2019, p. 1481).

Table 7.2: 'Core of steel' attributes (adapted from Hunt, 2019)

Key attribute	Characteristics
Solidarity	• Loyalty to their professional standards • Allegiance with patients' interests • Willingness to uphold shared values • Strong commitment to high-quality care • 'Buy-in' to the gatekeeping role
Tenacity	• Focused persistence • Perseverance in difficult circumstances • Would not relinquish their principles when under pressure • Prepared to 'fight to fail'
Audacity	• Bold and courageous • Willing to speak up to authority figures • Prepared to challenge convention • Handled opposition assertively • Undaunted when threatened
Integrity	• Worked to a clear, strong set of principles • Remained focused on what was right • Expectations did not fluctuate • Consistent in their decision-making
Dependability	• Composed and committed • Acknowledged their obligations • Made their meaning clear and unambiguous • Followed processes and procedures reliably • Resilient

Hunt (2019) argues that these criteria should be used to identify those individuals likely to be effective in the practice assessor role. Furthermore, Hunt goes on to suggest that practice supervisors and assessors require different qualities and personality traits. Practice supervisors are required to be nurturing, whereas practice assessors are less likely to inflate grades and are more exacting in their approach, and require a 'core of steel' (Hunt, 2019). Indeed, the paper challenges the NMC view that it is possible to act as both practice supervisor and assessor (albeit not to the same student) because the requirements of the roles are so different. The attributes listed in *Table 7.2* are offered as criteria for identifying potential practice assessors; Hunt draws on wider work to suggest that if organisations avoid doing this, then individuals could be appointed who may not be well aligned to the role, thus perpetuating 'failure to fail'.

7.8 SUMMARY

This chapter has provided an overview of the new practice assessor role, and responsibilities as set out by the standards for student supervision and assessment (NMC, 2018c). The chapter has provided some examples of assessment practices and outlined different types of assessment that could be used in clinical learning environments. The differences and benefits of formative and summative assessment have been described. Finally, the chapter has outlined the emotional aspects of assessing students in clinical practice. Throughout the chapter there are various activities which can also be used as evidence towards your revalidation activity to remain on the register.

RECOMMENDED FURTHER READING

LaDonna, K.A., Hatala, R., Lingard, L., Voyer, S. and Watling, C. (2017) Staging a performance: learners' perceptions about direct observation during residency. *Medical Education*, 51: 498–510.

Lamb, P.C. and Norton, C. (2018) Nurses experiences of using clinical competencies a qualitative study. *Nurse Education in Practice*, 31: 177–81.

Solheim, E., Syvertsen Plathe, H. and Eide, H. (2017) Nursing students' evaluation of a new feedback and reflection tool for use in high-fidelity simulation – Formative assessment of clinical skills. A descriptive quantitative research design. *Nurse Education in Practice*, 27: 114–20.

REFERENCES

Black, S., Curzio, J. and Terry, L. (2014) Failing a student nurse: A new horizon of moral courage. *Nursing Ethics*, **2(2)**: 224–38.

Boud, D. and Soler, R. (2016) Sustainable assessment revisited. *Assessment and Evaluation in Higher Education*, **41(3)**: 400–13. doi: 10.1080/02602938.2015.1018133

Cassidy, S. (2009) Subjectivity and the valid assessment of pre-registration student nurse clinical learning outcomes: Implications for mentors. *Nurse Education Today*, **29**: 33–9.

Cassidy, S., Coffey, M. and Murphy, F. (2017) 'Seeking authorization': a grounded theory exploration of mentors' experiences of assessing nursing students on the borderline of achievement of competence in clinical practice. *Journal of Advanced Nursing*, **73(9)**: 2167–78. doi: 10.1111/jan.13292

Duffy, K. (2003) Failing students: a qualitative study of factors that influence the decisions regarding assessment of students' competence in practice. Caledonian Nursing and Midwifery Research Centre School of Nursing, Midwifery and Community Health, Glasgow Caledonian University.

Duffy, K. and Hardicar, J. (2007) Supporting failing students in practice 1, assessment. *Nursing Times*, **103(47)**: 28–9.

Forber, J., DiGiacomo, M., Carter, B. *et al.* (2016) In pursuit of an optimal model of undergraduate nurse clinical education: An integrative review. *Nurse Education in Practice*, **21**: 83–92.

Happell, B. and Roper, C. (2010) The voice of experience: Consumer perspectives in the classroom. In: Warne, T. and McAndrew, S. (editors) *Creative Approaches to Health and Social Care Education*. Palgrave.

Health and Care Professions Council (2017) *Standards of education and training guidance*. HCPC. Available at: www.hcpc-uk.org/resources/guidance/standards-of-education-and-training-guidance/ (accessed 30 September 2020).

Helminen, K., Coco, K., Johnson, M., Turunen, H. and Tossavainen, K. (2016) Summative assessment of clinical practice of student nurses: A review of the literature. *International Journal of Nursing Studies*, **53**: 308–19.

Hughes, L.J., Johnston, A.N.B. and Mitchell, M.L. (2019) How organisational processes influence assessors' experiences of marginal students' performances in clinical assessments. *Collegian*, **26**: 242–9.

Hunt, L.A. (2019) Developing a 'core of steel': the key attributes of effective practice assessors. *British Journal of Nursing*, **28(22)**: 1478–84.

Hunt, L.A., McGee, P., Gutteridge, R. and Hughes, M. (2016) Manipulating mentors' assessment decisions: Do underperforming student nurses use coercive strategies to influence mentors' practical assessment decisions? *Nurse Education in Practice*, **20**: 154–62. doi: 10.1016/j.nepr.2016.08.007

Kajander-Unkuri, S., Leino-Kilpi, H., Katajisto, J. *et al.* (2016) Congruence between graduating nursing students' self-assessments and mentors' assessments of students' nurse competence. *Collegian*, **23**: 303–12.

Leigh, J. and Roberts, D. (2018) Critical exploration of the new NMC standards of proficiency for registered nurses. *British Journal of Nursing*, **27(18)**: 1068–72.

Levett-Jones, T., Gersbach, J., Arthur, C. and Roche, J. (2011) Implementing a clinical competency assessment model that promotes critical reflection and ensures nursing graduates' readiness for professional practice. *Nurse Education in Practice*, **11**: 64–9.

McSherry, R. and Duggan, S. (2016) Involving carers in the teaching, learning and assessment of masters students. *Nurse Education in Practice*, **16**: 156–9.

Nursing and Midwifery Council (2018a) *Future nurse: Standards of proficiency for registered nurses*. NMC. Available at: www.nmc.org.uk/globalassets/sitedocuments/education-standards/future-nurse-proficiencies.pdf (accessed 17 August 2020).

Nursing and Midwifery Council (2018b) *Realising professionalism: Part 1: Standards framework for nursing and midwifery education*. NMC. Available at: www.nmc.org.uk/globalassets/sitedocuments/education-standards/education-framework.pdf (accessed 13 August 2020).

Nursing and Midwifery Council (2018c) *Realising professionalism: Part 2: Standards for student supervision and assessment*. NMC. Available at: www.nmc.org.uk/globalassets/sitedocuments/education-standards/student-supervision-assessment.pdf (accessed 13 August 2020).

Open University (2020) *Facilitating learning in practice: Types of assessment*. Available at: www.open.edu/openlearn/ocw/mod/oucontent/view.php?id=20113&section=2 (accessed 28 September 2020).

Roberts, D. (2011) Grading the performance of clinical skills: Lessons to be learned from the performing arts. *Nurse Education Today*, **31(6)**: 607–10.

Speers, J. and Lathlean, J. (2015) Service user involvement in giving mental health students feedback on placement: A participatory action research study. *Nurse Education Today*, 35(9): 84–9.

Warne, T. and McAndrew, S. (editors) (2004) *Using patient experience in nurse education*. Palgrave.

Zasadny, M.F. and Bull, R.M. (2015) Assessing competence in undergraduate nursing students: The Amalgamated Students Assessment in Practice model. *Nurse Education in Practice*, 15: 126–33.

ACTIVITY ANSWER GUIDES

ACTIVITY 7.2

The questions posed here might make you think of a range of knowledge and skills that you would expect the student to demonstrate; these are effectively the criteria that you will use to make a judgement about whether the student is proficient in this area of practice. For example, you might have considered:

- Effective communication skills with the patient and the family
- Assessment of physical needs; for example pain relief, management of urinary waste (retention of urine, renal failure and/or catheterisation)
- Psychological assessment and management of anxiety of the patient and family members.

ACTIVITY 7.3

In relation to the following NMC outcome statement:

Examples in relation to specific NMC standards include the following: "1.16: Demonstrate the ability to keep complete, clear, accurate and timely records"; you might want to consider whether you expect the student to do this once, most of the time or all of the time right from the start of the programme, or by the time they are in part 2 of the programme? You should also discuss your thoughts with other assessors to ensure that you are providing a consistent approach.

If it is a more generic proficiency such as: "5.6: Exhibit leadership potential by demonstrating an ability to guide, support and motivate individuals and interact confidently with other members of the care team"; is there a similar continuum here or is there something in your mind that would constitute a 'pass' for this outcome? Are your thoughts similar or different to those of other practice assessors in your area?

CHAPTER 8

USING SIMULATION-BASED EDUCATION FOR SUPERVISION AND ASSESSMENT OF STUDENT LEARNING

Leah Greene

8.1 INTRODUCTION

This chapter will provide an overview of the range of healthcare simulation from procedural to immersive simulation and will discuss the benefits of enabling students to learn in a safe, supportive, simulated environment. Nursing and Midwifery Council (NMC) *Part 1: Standards framework for nursing and midwifery education* (NMC, 2018b, p. 9, 3.4) states: "Approved education institutions, together with practice learning partners, must ensure that all students are enabled to learn and are assessed using a range of methods, including technology enhanced and simulation-based learning appropriate for their programme as necessary for safe and effective practice". Therefore, as practice supervisors and assessors it is important that you understand the theory behind how to use simulation effectively in clinical practice; and then go on to apply the principles to the area where you work.

After reading this chapter you will be able to:
- Describe a range of approaches to simulation in healthcare
- Identify a range of situations that are common where you work where simulation could be used
- Work with colleagues to devise and develop relevant scenarios for learners to experience.

8.2 BACKGROUND

There is a tendency to think that simulation is new, but for over a century simulation has been used in medical and healthcare education, in the form of anatomical models, task trainers and role-play (Nehring and Lashley, 2009). The first life-sized manikin, Mrs Chase, was produced in 1911 for practising clinical nursing skills in Hartford Hospital Training School in Connecticut (Herrmann, 1981). Mrs Chase, the first 'proxy patient', enabled nursing students to practise skills without "inconveniencing or harming patients" (Grypma, 2012, p. 181). Baby demonstration dolls were also developed and produced in 1913 for midwifery skills practice (Herrmann, 1981). These life-size manikins gained popularity in the 1950s and 1960s when users realised that they helped students put theories into practice (Hyland and Hawkins, 2009; Roberts and Greene, 2011). Over the last 50 years, the use of simulation and technology in nursing education has developed significantly. Innovative technologies, such as e-learning and simulation now enhance traditional teaching and learning techniques, allowing the health and social care workforce to rehearse skills and train more flexibly (Department of Health, 2011).

8.2.1 Different types of simulation

Often simulation can be seen as related only to the technology involved to enable the realisation of clinical scenarios. Gaba's definition of simulation, however, explains that simulation is:

> "a technique, not a technology, to replace or amplify real experiences with guided experiences, often immersive in nature, that evoke or replicate substantial aspects of the real world in a fully interactive fashion". (Gaba, 2004, p. i2)

In fact, there is a broad spectrum of simulation (Purva *et al.*, 2016). At one end of the spectrum are case studies and role-play, techniques used to educate healthcare professionals for centuries. Procedural simulation, which can be defined as "the use of a simulation modality (e.g. task trainer, manikin, computer) to assist in the process of learning to complete a technical skill, or a procedure" (International Nursing Association for Clinical Simulation and Learning (INACSL) Standards Committee, 2016b, pp. S43–44) would feature further along the spectrum. At the other end, you would find fully immersive simulation-based experiences, which comprise "a broad array of structured activities that represent actual or potential situations in education, practice and research" (INACSL Standards Committee, 2016b, p. S45). Immersive simulation is designed to allow learners to develop or enhance knowledge, skills and attitudes in a safe environment while responding to realistic situations. Gaba (2004) describes a "rich and complex tapestry of simulation" and refers to 11 dimensions, that can be used to categorise simulation activities in healthcare education; some of these will be discussed briefly later in the chapter. *Figure 8.1* illustrates the spectrum of simulation.

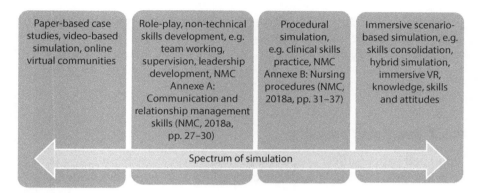

| Paper-based case studies, video-based simulation, online virtual communities | Role-play, non-technical skills development, e.g. team working, supervision, leadership development, NMC Annexe A: Communication and relationship management skills (NMC, 2018a, pp. 27–30) | Procedural simulation, e.g. clinical skills practice, NMC Annexe B: Nursing procedures (NMC, 2018a, pp. 31–37) | Immersive scenario-based simulation, e.g. skills consolidation, hybrid simulation, immersive VR, knowledge, skills and attitudes |

Spectrum of simulation

Figure 8.1: *Spectrum of simulation.*

When choosing the simulation modality, first and foremost you must consider the learning objectives: what are the learners there to learn? Once the learning objectives have been defined, the teaching methods and simulation modality can be clarified. It is very important that the pedagogy leads the use of simulation, rather than the technology (Roberts and Greene, 2011). Or to be more specific, rather than pedagogy, it must be the andragogy, the method and practice of teaching adult learners, which should guide the selection of simulation modality. For example, it is not necessary to place learners into an immersive simulation environment if they are learning an individual skill for the first time; this would be far too distracting and overwhelming for the learner. Practical clinical skills can, and should, be practised in a safe, low-risk or classroom environment using task trainers and simple manikins alone prior to learners combining multiple clinical skills and/or non-psychomotor skills. If the learning objective is to practise non-psychomotor skills, e.g. communication, leadership or team-working skills, then role-play would be the most beneficial modality. Once the learners have practised and acquired the required skills, they can then be consolidated in an immersive scenario-based simulation. Immersive simulation can involve simulated patients, computer-controlled high-tech manikins that exhibit signs and signals and/or hybrid simulation, where task trainers are linked to a simulated patient (Lioce *et al.*, 2020).

☑ **ACTIVITY 8.1**

Before moving on as a practice supervisor or assessor start to think about the clinical and non-psychomotor skills that students might need to learn while they are working alongside you: how might you incorporate some low-risk simulation into the students' learning?

Are there some psychomotor skills that you think students should already have before they are placed in your area; and how might they gain these skills?

An answer guide is provided at the end of this chapter.

8.2.2 Simulated patients

Simulated patients (SPs) are people trained to consistently portray a patient or other individual in a scripted scenario for the purposes of instruction, practice or evaluation (INACSL Standards Committee, 2016b, p. S45). SPs also portray the roles of relatives, carers, trainee healthcare students and qualified healthcare professionals (Nestel *et al.*, 2010). SPs may participate in teaching and assessment and provide feedback to learners. They have particular value in providing feedback on issues relevant to patient-centredness. Due to the realistic and interactive nature of immersive simulation, it is possible to practise both clinical and non-technical skills in environments where learners are supported, enabled and encouraged to make decisions and take actions in a safe learning environment that represents realistic healthcare situations (Lioce *et al.*, 2020). *Scenario 8.3*, later in this chapter, provides an overview of an immersive, dynamic, interprofessional simulation with embedded SPs, high-tech manikin patients, simulated patient relatives and simulated healthcare professionals. This type of simulation can be used to facilitate the transition from pre-registration student to newly qualified staff nurse, as learners are given the opportunity to practise both clinical and non-psychomotor skills and the principles of human factors (see *Recommended further reading*) in a safe, supportive environment enabling them to become 'supervisor ready' graduates of the future as outlined in NMC (2018a) *Future nurse: Standards of proficiency for registered nurses*:

> "*5.8: support and supervise students in the delivery of nursing care, promoting reflection and providing constructive feedback, and evaluating and documenting their performance*
>
> *5.9: demonstrate the ability to challenge and provide constructive feedback about care delivered by others in the*

team, and support them to identify and agree individual learning needs

    5.10: contribute to supervision and team reflection activities to promote improvements in practice and services".

☑ ACTIVITY 8.2

Download the *Healthcare Simulation Dictionary* (2nd edition): www.ahrq.gov/sites/default/files/wysiwyg/patient-safety/resources/simulation/sim-dictionary-2nd.pdf
    Consider the different modalities of simulation. What types of simulation have you been involved in previously, either as a pre-registration or post-registration learner or facilitator? How could you incorporate some of this within your work as a practice supervisor or assessor?
    This is a personal reflective activity, so no answer guide is provided.

8.3 TECHNOLOGY-ENHANCED LEARNING

Recent advances in technology have indicated a shift in the way the future NHS workforce will interact with patients, claiming that genomics, digital medicine, artificial intelligence (AI) and robotics will change the role and function of clinical staff over the next 20 years (Topol, 2019). Topol (2019) further states that four of the top ten digital healthcare technologies that will impact on current models of care are:
- Telemedicine
- Smartphone apps
- Sensors and wearables for diagnostics and remote monitoring
- Virtual reality (VR) and augmented reality (AR).

These disruptive technologies will directly impact the future health and social care workforce. As a result, educators, including practice supervisors and assessors, have a responsibility to fully prepare learners to enable them to confidently perform in this changing digital world (NMC, 2018a, p. 20, 5.11: "effectively and responsibly use a range of digital technologies to access, input, share and apply information and data within teams and between agencies"). VR emerged in the 1960s with Ivan Sutherland's 'Sword of Damocles' (Sutherland, 1968), the first system to use computer-generated graphics in a head-mounted display. It even had cutting-edge features such as head tracking, which made it more immersive than any other system at the time. However, it also had limitations; it was so heavy that it had to be suspended from the ceiling by an adjustable pole.

ACTIVITY 8.3

If you are not familiar with virtual reality, watch this short YouTube clip to view an example of the first VR headset:
www.youtube.com/watch?v=NtwZXGprxag

No answer guide is required for this activity.

8.3.1 *Computer-based simulation*

Computer-based simulation, including virtual patients, VR task trainers and immersive VR simulation, is becoming more common in healthcare education. In 2004, Gaba predicted that a variety of technologies will be relevant for simulation in the future. Nowadays, different simulation modalities, such as video-based, virtual, remote and online simulation (Lioce *et al.*, 2020), are accepted methods used for teaching and learning, in particular, non-technical skills. Gaba (2004) also commented that complex tasks and experiences can be recreated using technology, and some education and training on teamwork can be accomplished using videos. To highlight this further, Gaba (2004) also explains one of the benefits of using videos, computer programs or the internet for simulation is that it can be experienced wherever the learner is situated, using a personal computer or other device.

Second Life® (SL) is an online virtual world created by Linden Lab and launched in 2003 (Linden Research, Inc., 2019). Virtual worlds like SL differ from traditional computer games as they do not have a specific goal or end-point; they have a social context and multiple users engage with each other to take part in social activities or educational opportunities (Aebersold *et al.*, 2012). While the SL platform and its graphics are not classified as advanced, users report that the environment is "acceptable for role play and simulations involving interpersonal interactions" (Aebersold *et al.*, 2012, e471). Some learners have even stated that the experience with SL was "better than or as good as SimMan®", a high-tech simulation manikin (Aebersold *et al.*, 2012, p. e473). Examples of scenarios that have been developed in SL are family health, disaster preparedness and home safety (Schaffer *et al.*, 2016), and safety issues with adverse events, difficult interprofessional communications and priority setting (Aebersold *et al.*, 2012). Research has demonstrated that SL is an effective platform for the development of virtual simulation-based learning experiences that are transferrable to real world clinical practice (Aebersold *et al.*, 2012; Benham-Hutchins and Lall, 2015; Tiffany and Hoglund, 2014; Schaffer *et al.*, 2016; Walia *et al.*, 2017). Due to the nature of SL, multiple users can interact in the same time and space, which is useful for collaboration, immersive role-playing and real-time interaction including the possibility of using SL for a virtual post-simulation debrief environment for multiple participants.

In addition to video-based simulation, online virtual worlds and physical simulation activities, learners can also benefit from accessing virtual communities. Here they explore the complexity of individuals and families; the people and places they encounter help learners to apply complex context to theoretical components of their programmes. In the virtual community, learners meet virtual simulated patients and relatives prior to interacting with them during physical simulation-based experiences. As the virtual community is online, learners are able to access the content whenever and wherever they like as a pre-brief prior to simulation sessions or as a recap following on from simulation post debrief.

8.3.2 *An example of using a virtual community in supervision and assessment*

Birley Place is a virtual community (Greene *et al.*, 2020) available for all students in the Faculty of Health, Psychology and Social Care at Manchester Metropolitan University (Manchester Met), UK. Birley Place uses a blended learning approach to enable students to participate in virtual simulation, interprofessional education (IPE), group and independent study. The realistic cases, scenarios, people and places encountered in Birley Place allow learners to explore the complexity of individuals and families within the context of the profession they are studying see (https://birleyplace.mmu.ac.uk/). All of the simulated people in Birley Place have an associated SP role profile (discussed briefly later in this chapter). In addition to the homes within the virtual community there are also shared spaces; for example, a hospital, health centre, parks, leisure centres, primary and secondary schools, shops, restaurants and a police station. An example of one of the virtual people featured in Birley Place is Anthony James (see *Figure 8.2*).

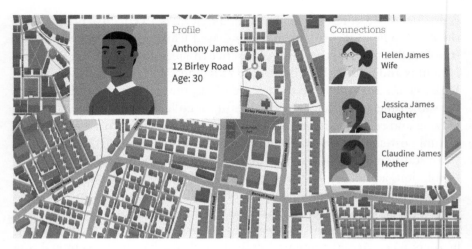

Figure 8.2: *Example of Birley Place map and SP profile; reproduced with permission ©Manchester Metropolitan University, 2019; all rights reserved.*

📂 **SCENARIO 8.1**

Profile: Anthony James

Anthony lives at No. 12 Birley Road with his wife Helen and their daughter Jessica. Jessica attends Gaskell Lane Primary School. Anthony has a brother, Paul, who lives in Liverpool and a mother, Claudine, who lives nearby in Flat 20, 136 Bonsall Road. Anthony's father died a year ago from cancer although his mother and father divorced several years earlier. Anthony is self-employed and runs a small advertising company. He is fit and active and loves riding his motorbike. He is also involved in a number of sports including five-a-side football and martial arts. Helen is a care assistant and works at Sunshine House Nursing Home. Anthony and Helen have been married for 6 years. Helen's parents live in Scotland and she does not see them often, so she relies on her mother-in-law, Claudine, for assistance with childcare.

Anthony and his family feature in multiple scenarios throughout the nursing and physiotherapy programmes at Manchester Met in virtual simulation, case-based interprofessional education and during fully immersive physical simulation. For example, Anthony is brought to the trauma room via paramedic transfer during a second-year pre-registration student nurse trauma simulation. He has been involved in a road traffic accident on his motorbike. He has a fractured pelvis, fractured tibia and fibula, left haemothorax and significant brain injury. Anthony is treated during the trauma simulation and the scenario concludes as he is taken for a computed tomography (CT) scan. Helen also enters the scenario as a concerned relative. Anthony's scenario continues in the weeks following his accident with interprofessional linked learning activities with second-year nursing students learning from and with second-year physiotherapy students regarding his physical rehabilitation post-surgery, and mental health nursing students to discuss Anthony's psychological recovery. Aspects of his home life feature in these discussions, including reference to his work, family and financial status, thereby creating a holistic, realistic, sequential simulation experience for the learners.

You can see here how *Scenario 8.1* is true to life and reflects a typical patient journey. The scenario includes learning and teaching opportunities as the learner interacts with others in the scenario, including people from other professions.

8.4 WRITING EFFECTIVE SCENARIOS

As previously mentioned, the key to ensuring effective learning during simulation is defining achievable learning objectives from the outset. By using well designed and constructed scenarios, you can ensure that the learners, facilitators, simulated patients and technical colleagues are properly prepared and supported throughout the simulation from induction, to pre-brief and beyond the scenario itself during the debrief and post-event reflection activities. Frameworks and proformas exist to assist with scenario design, one of which is described here:

The integrated simulation and technology enhanced learning (ISTEL) framework (Gough *et al.*, 2016a, b; Nestel and Gough, 2018) integrates three distinct but interlinking essential components, which should be considered when designing, developing, implementing, evaluating or researching simulation and technology enhanced learning (STEL). These are *preparation*, *intervention* and *evaluation/research*. These three components are further subdivided into eight elements:

1 Learner; 2 Facilitator; 3 Theory and educational practices; 4 Learning design characteristics; 5 Pre-brief and debrief; 6 Linked learning activities; 7 Outcomes; and 8 Economic evaluation.

The ISTEL framework can be used as a guide to enable users to properly prepare to undertake simulation-based education:

> "*The ISTEL framework emphasizes the importance of ensuring appropriate theoretical and educational practices underpin the design, preparation, implementation and evaluation of STEL interventions; whether this be for a scenario, short course or embedded within healthcare curricula*". (Gough *et al.*, 2016a, e28).

TOP TIP

These elements could also be applied to any extended learning activity, not just those involving simulation.

Consider *Scenario 8.2* as an example of how the ISTEL framework can be utilised to plan a very basic simulation-based experience.

SCENARIO 8.2

You must teach first-year nursing and midwifery students hand hygiene techniques. You need to prepare the students to be assessed on the following outcome statements: NMC *Future nurse: Standards of proficiency for registered nurses*: Annexe B: *Nursing procedures*, section 9: "Use evidence-based, best practice approaches for meeting needs for care and support with the prevention and management of infection, accurately assessing the person's capacity for independence and self-care and initiating appropriate interventions"; subsection 9.6: "Use evidence-based hand hygiene techniques" (NMC, 2018a, p. 36).

How could you use the ISTEL framework to guide this session while in clinical practice?

Using the headings from the ISTEL framework as a guide, the learning can be mapped out as follows:

1. **Learners** Multiprofessional, first-year nursing and/or midwifery students
2. **Facilitator** Practice supervisor/nurse academics
3. **Theories and educational practices** Behaviourism (Skinner, 1938), deliberate practice (Ericsson *et al.*, 1993), experiential learning (Kolb, 1984).
4. **Learning design characteristics**

Learning objectives:
- to understand the role of hand hygiene in preventing the spread of infection
- to select the appropriate hand hygiene method
- to perform the correct steps required for hand washing and applying alcohol gel
- to identify when hand hygiene is required.

Design – modality required is procedural simulation of hand hygiene skills in an appropriate environment; in this case with hospital-style sinks, liquid soap, paper towels and hand gel. But if you were working in a community setting in someone's home, your environment would be different and should be taken into account.

Fidelity, realism and authenticity – environment and equipment should be realistic and represent a clinical setting to ensure repeatability, replicability and buy-in from learners.

📁 **SCENARIO 8.2**   *(cont'd)*

5. **Pre-brief and debrief** Beforehand, learners should be sent the '7 steps of hand washing' guide, a link to the hand washing practice video and the hand washing assessment criteria to enable them to properly prepare for the session and ascertain the steps required to be classed as proficient. You might think that this is knowledge that the learner should have before attending your placement. You might also think about giving the student ample opportunities to rehearse the skill and provide them with feedback and feedforward advice.

Following the session, during an informal debrief or feedback session learners should be given the opportunity to reflect on their skills in relation to the learning objectives, using these questions as a prompt:
- How can hand hygiene prevent the spread of infection?
- Can you tell me which hand hygiene method you would select in this situation?
- Talk me though the seven steps required for hand washing and applying alcohol gel
- Can you give me examples of when hand hygiene is required?

These questions can be asked by the practice supervisor or assessor to check knowledge and understanding, and application of theory to practice.
6. **Linked learning activities** Following reflection, opportunities for further practice sessions and linked learning should be issued to the learners. For example, ask the learners to consider how this scenario could be adapted if they were working in the community and had to undertake a wound dressing in someone's home?
7. **Outcomes** Following this session, learners should be equipped with the knowledge, skills, attitudes and behaviours required to perform effective hand hygiene. Learners should understand the rationale behind hand hygiene to prevent the spread of infection and the translation of this knowledge into practice prior to clinical placement.
8. **Economic evaluation** Consider the true cost of this simple scenario, e.g. staffing, consumables, facilities, training and time required. Could it be delivered in a more cost-effective manner?

Another example of a framework that can be used to aid the design of effective scenarios is the INACSL standards of best practice, which outline 11 criteria for effective 'simulation design'. They state that simulation-based experiences should be designed to meet identified learning objectives, which will optimise the achievement of expected outcomes and, as a result, strengthen the overall value of the simulation-based experience (INACSL Standards Committee, 2016a). The 11 criteria for simulation design are depicted in *Figure 8.3*.

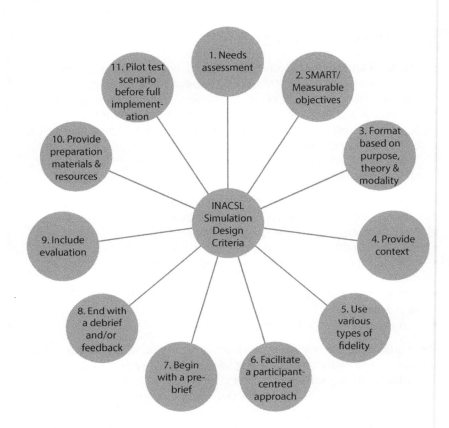

Figure 8.3: *INACSL criteria for effective simulation design (INACSL, 2016a).*

The 11 INACSL simulation design criteria can be adapted to provide a practical template or checklist to ensure that simulation is well designed.

☑ ACTIVITY 8.4

Review the INACSL standard for simulation design:
www.inacsl.org/inacsl-standards-of-best-practice-simulation/

Produce a template as an example. Consider scenarios you have designed or participated in: how do they compare with the required elements of the 11 INACSL criteria necessary to meet this standard? Think about how you might use these criteria to help you (and your colleagues) to develop scenarios to support clinical learning against some of the NMC (2018a) *Future nurse* standard outcome statements that are relevant to the area or service where you work.

This is a personal reflective activity, so no answer guide is provided.

Evidence-based scenario design templates such as these provided here are available to help you to standardise the design process and ensure quality of the materials produced, irrespective of the simulation modality whether this be for video-based simulation, role-play, procedural or immersive simulation.

In the North West of England, there is a scenario library of over 200 peer-reviewed scenarios and a supportive culture of mentoring and sharing best practice in the region. Members of the North West Simulation Education Network (NWSEN) also have access to e-learning and face-to-face training and an accreditation programme provided by NWSEN and supported by Health Education England (HEE). The NWSEN scenario design 'simulation proforma' template guides the user through the essential steps to enable them to produce effective simulation scenarios. Once designed on the proforma, scenarios can then be submitted for peer review and uploaded onto the shared scenario library. The proforma also includes a statement on mental health for users to consider:

> *"It is important that we actively consider the mental health aspects of our patients, as well as the physical health ones, and include these aspects in the scenario development process. As a result, there is now a 'mental health state' in the timeline to demonstrate changes and key points; we would encourage you to consider these and work with mental health colleagues to include this element".* (NWSEN, 2016, p. 3)

In addition to the mental health aspects, the proforma includes sections for the following, which must be completed to ensure the scenario is correctly designed:

- Overall goals
- Learning objectives
- Faculty requirements
- Participant information
- Brief summary
- Simulation equipment requirements
- Set up overview
- Patient demographics
- Medical equipment requirements
- Scenario handover information
- Timeline overview (including both physical and mental health aspects, expected actions and prompts required for each stage)
- Key debrief points linked to the learning objectives

- Key message slides/handouts
- Simulated patient information (as an appendix)
- Additional supportive educational material and references.

8.5 BEING 'SUPERVISOR READY'

It is the responsibility of higher education institutions and practice placements to ensure that all students have the opportunity to collaborate with each other, participate in IPE and develop both clinical and non-technical skills. According to the NMC, all students must:

> *"have opportunities throughout their programme to collaborate and learn with and from other professionals, to learn with and from peers, and to develop supervision and leadership skills".*
> (NMC, 2018b, p. 10)

Simulation-based education (SBE) offers opportunities for learners to collaborate with peers, both uniprofessionally (meaning as a single profession) and interprofessionally (meaning with other professional groups). By physically participating in SBE and observing peers vicariously, learners can make sense of the scenario by being fully engaged in the situation and by participating in active listening and reflective thinking (Roberts, 2010; Roberts and Greene, 2011). In this way, students are learning and thinking together. This process is further enhanced during simulation debrief where both active participants and vicarious learners participate in a structured, facilitated discussion and are encouraged to reflect together on the scenario that previously took place. As a practice supervisor you might want to pair third-year students with first- or second-year students and ask them to facilitate learning and provide feedback for that student as part of their preparation to be supervisor ready.

Similarly, SBE allows students the opportunity to develop non-technical leadership and management skills outlined in *Future nurse: Standards of proficiency for registered nurses*, Annexe A (NMC, 2018a). By establishing well-designed simulation scenarios, students can practise communication skills with patients, families and carers, peers and professional teams. While we would not ordinarily encourage student learners to 'act-up' to a higher level than the level that they are studying, when students are about to qualify, SBE can be integrated into the curriculum to enable them to take on the role of a newly qualified staff nurse, while being fully supported during the simulation and with the opportunity for post-event reflection and debrief. *Scenario 8.3* summarises an interprofessional, continuous, sequential simulation designed for soon-to-be-qualified third-year student nurses. During the simulation and subsequent debrief, post-event reflection and linked learning activities, students are encouraged to practise, refine and reflect on their communication, decision-making, leadership and management skills, thereby promoting the essential skills required for students to become new registrants who are 'supervisor ready' upon qualification.

 SCENARIO 8.3

Staff nurse toolkit (SNT) (Borneuf and Rickels, 2016)

The SNT will now be discussed to give an example of how immersive simulation can be used as a technique to develop students' supervision and leadership skills. Variations of the SNT on a smaller scale involving fewer simulated patients, relatives and colleagues could be considered to achieve similar learning objectives in clinical practice. As a team of practice supervisors and assessors you might be able to adapt this approach.

Overall goals The purpose of the SNT is to enable the student to apply skills of critical analysis to real world situations to support the transition from student to newly qualified nurse.

Learning objectives:

1. Critically appraise the process of identifying clinical priorities within a fluctuating healthcare environment to maintain patient safety. NMC, 2018a, 20, 5.5: "safely and effectively lead and manage the nursing care of a group of people, demonstrating appropriate prioritisation, delegation and assignment of care responsibilities to others involved in providing care"; 5.6: "exhibit leadership potential by demonstrating an ability to guide, support and motivate individuals and interact confidently with other members of the care team".

2. Demonstrate application of effective team working and leadership skills to safely manage patient care. NMC, 2018a, 20, 5.1: "understand the principles of effective leadership, management, group and organisational dynamics and culture and apply these to team working and decision-making"; 5.2: "understand and apply the principles of human factors, environmental factors and strength-based approaches when working in teams"; 5.3: "understand the principles and application of processes for performance management and how these apply to the nursing team"; 5.4: "demonstrate an understanding of the roles, responsibilities and scope of practice of all members of the nursing and interdisciplinary team and how to make best use of the contributions of others involved in providing care".

3. Deploy communication strategies to effectively manage varying clinical situations to achieve high-quality patient care.

4. Critically evaluate a simulated clinical environment to identify the legal, professional and ethical perspectives encountered.

📁 **SCENARIO 8.3**　　　*(cont'd)*

Faculty requirements The SNT is a dynamic, immersive simulation involving four high-tech computer-controlled manikin patients, three human SPs, two simulated healthcare professionals, three simulated relatives and an embedded facilitator. If you were developing this scenario for use in practice you would need to think about this in relation to the requirements in your context.

Participant information The SNT is designed for third-year student nurses who are soon to qualify. However, it would be appropriate to include other student healthcare professionals and associated practice supervisors in an interprofessional team simulation, e.g. student physiotherapists, speech and language therapists, occupational therapists, radiographers, social workers, etc.

Brief summary The SNT is designed to simulate 2 hours of a shift on a busy mixed surgical assessment ward. The ward has two bays of patients and two side-rooms. There will be patients on the ward who are under the care of medical consultants. They are on the ward due to 'bed pressures'. Learners will be expected to carry out necessary duties and respond to patient needs. The clinical environment will give third-year students the opportunity to practise and refine skills including, but not restricted to:

- Communication
- Leadership
- Management
- Prioritisation skills
- Delegation
- Team working
- Conflict resolution
- Risk management/assessment
- Resilience.

The SNT is a full-day three-stage continuous teaching and learning activity. Three groups of approximately 15 pre-registration nursing students participate in different stages of this continuous scenario (15 students per group identified as SNT1, SNT2, SNT3). Students engage in activities that will allow them to safely operate in the role of a registered nurse. The experience is consolidated immediately following each group's 2-hour scenario, and then in-depth during a facilitated post-event reflection and debrief the following day. If delivering this scenario in clinical practice you would need to think about the area where the simulation will take place, the time span that each learner is expected to spend in the scenario, and availability of others.

Simulation equipment requirements Various equipment is required to create a realistic and authentic simulation experience including, for example, clinical record folders and inserts for all patients, medical notes trolley, desk for ward clerk, telephone, observation equipment, medicines trolley, drugs charts, controlled drugs (CDs) cupboard, CD book, resuscitation trolley, moving and handling equipment including hoist, nebuliser, oxygen masks, syringe driver,

SCENARIO 8.3   *(cont'd)*

clock, patient wrist bands, theatre gowns, pen torches, glucometer, urinalysis equipment, vomit bowls, fluid balance charts, IV saline, giving sets and so on. You can adapt the equipment list to suit your environment, but you might want to consider aspects such as shortage of certain equipment or having to locate equipment within the area.

Set up overview Two side-rooms (SR1 and SR2), two ward bays, one clean utility, one store room.

Patient demographics Within the toolkit all patient roles are designed using SP role profile documentation (for more information on role profile development, see *Recommended further reading* and Gough and Greene, 2015; Gough, Greene, Nestel *et al.*, 2015; and Greene and Gough, 2016). This includes rich information about each simulated patient, simulated relative and simulated healthcare professional to enable the person carrying out the role to provide a holistic detailed performance. The SP role describes the 'person elements' of the SP role. The 'learning activity' is described next, followed by the 'context' and any other considerations for the role, including clothing, special effects make-up (moulage) and any props required (Greene and Gough, 2016).

Scenario handover information Handover is given to all learners for each stage of the SNT using the situation, background, assessment, recommendation (SBAR) communication tool (Müller *et al.*, 2018; Stewart and Hand, 2017). Students are also given a blank 'handover sheet' with the patient details (room/bay number, patient name, NHS number and date of birth). The handover sheet also has space for them to make notes and write any actions during handover.

Timeline overview A detailed timeline of events, including both physical and mental health aspects, expected actions and prompts required for each stage, is included for each of the seven patient scenarios (both human SP and manikin patient). As the SNT is an immersive, dynamic simulation, designed for large groups of learners, timelines often cross with multiple events and activities occurring simultaneously. Learners are expected to manage their time effectively and identify key clinical priorities, while working as a team.

 TOP TIP

In clinical practice, you could develop the role profiles to mirror your patient population. You might want to think about whether there are staff colleagues who could perform these roles or perhaps patient engagement groups?

Key debrief points There are four elements to the SNT debrief as follows:

Element 1 An immediate post-event debrief using the SHARP tool (Ahmed *et al.*, 2013; Arora *et al.*, 2012) to guide the debrief directly linked to the session learning objectives. The immediacy of this debrief optimises learning. Learners are asked to consider the following:

- How did it go? What went well and why?
- Address concerns: what did not go well and why?
- Review of learning points. Were your learning objectives met? What did you learn about your management and leadership skills? What did you learn about your team working skills?
- Plan ahead. What actions can you take to improve your practice? (Arora *et al.*, 2012).

Element 2 Students are required to review their own learning objectives to consider whether these were achieved during the simulation. From this, they will identify their developmental needs analysis based on reflections on their own practice to inform their learning as they transition into the staff nurse role. This activity occurs as timetabled directed study the following morning.

Element 3 The Diamond debrief tool (Jaye *et al.*, 2015) is then utilised to guide a large group debrief activity to facilitate triangulation of learning and reflection between and within groups. Information generated from elements 1 and 2 informs the debrief. This enables the students to describe their experience as a group focusing on a description of what happened, analysis phase and application of learning (Jaye *et al.*, 2015). During analysis learners examine their thoughts, feelings, attitudes and knowledge to 'unpack' *why* they did what they did and *what* influenced them in making the decisions they made. The final phase of the Diamond debrief will consider the application of their learning, to include the consideration of alternative situations, what they will do differently in the future and how the skills required to manage the SNT can be developed.

Element 4 An evaluation of the SNT activity takes place via a virtual learning environment, e.g. Moodle or Blackboard, to inform the facilitators about any improvements or changes required that can be integrated to enhance future learning opportunities for subsequent learners undertaking future immersive simulation.

Debriefing is an important skill for all practice supervisors. Being aware of frameworks and models such as the ones provided here can be helpful to ensure that you support the students to maximise the learning from any clinical situation (whether simulated or real).

📝 **ACTIVITY 8.5**

As a practice supervisor you could start to plan how you can use this debriefing approach at the end of an episode of care.

This is a personal reflective activity, so no answer guide is provided.

8.6 USING SIMULATION FOR ASSESSMENTS

SBE can be used as a technique to facilitate formative assessments, summative assessments and objective structured clinical examinations (OSCEs). Formative assessments are assessments *for* learning whereas summative assessments are assessments *of* learning (Gough and Greene, 2016). OSCEs are a station or series of stations designed to assess performance competency or other professional skills (Lioce *et al.*, 2020). SPs are routinely embedded into assessments and OSCEs as 'human examination questions' (Nestel and Bearman, 2015; Smith *et al.*, 2015). Involving SPs in assessments allows examiners the opportunity to offer the learners a realistic, interactive patient-centred experience (Gough and Greene, 2016). In the same way that SP role profiles must be designed for immersive SBE, they should be developed in the same way for OSCEs to enable an effective and often standardised performance for all examination candidates.

There are resource, recruitment and selection, training, risk assessment, ethical and quality assurance considerations associated with involving SPs in assessments. The elements of the SP common framework and checklist (Gough and Greene, 2015; Gough *et al.*, 2015) provide guidance for anyone involving SPs in SBE or assessments. To overcome any issues associated with the five elements of the SP common framework, alternative simulation modalities from the spectrum of simulation (see *Figure 8.1*) can be employed to deliver effective virtual or video-based simulation.

8.7 SUMMARY

This chapter has introduced a broad spectrum of simulation and discussion around different simulation modalities that can be used for a range of SBE activities; the key point to remember is that they are all valid techniques, but the modality must be appropriate and linked to the learning objectives. Innovative technology and creative content including video-based simulation, virtual and augmented reality and virtual communities are finding momentum and will directly impact the future health and social care workforce and need to be embraced in this changing digital world. Writing effective, top-quality scenarios and role profiles, which can be overlaid onto human SPs, manikins or virtual patients, creates a realistic, authentic experience for the learners. Examples have been given to highlight useful frameworks, proformas and areas of best practice that currently exist to enable learners to get the most out of SBE, which in turn prepares them for their future career in healthcare.

RECOMMENDED FURTHER READING

Gough, S., Greene, L., Natali, A. *et al.* (2016) Increasing the quality and value of involving simulated patients in simulation-based education, research and practice. *Physiotherapy*, **102**: e225–6.

Kneebone, R. (2016) Simulation reframed. *Advances in Simulation*, **1**: 27. doi: 10.1186/s41077-016-0028-8

Lavelle, M., Attoeb, C., Tritschlerb, C. and Cross, S. (2017) Managing medical emergencies in mental health settings using an interprofessional in-situ simulation training programme: A mixed methods evaluation study. *Nurse Education Today*, **59**: 103–9.

Syed, M. (2015) *Black box thinking*. John Murray.

REFERENCES

Aebersold, M., Tschannen, D., Stephens, M., Anderson, P. and Lei, X. (2012) Second Life®: A new strategy in educating nursing students. *Clinical Simulation in Nursing*, **8(9)**: e469–75.

Ahmed, M., Arora, S., Russ, S. *et al.* (2013) Operation debrief: a SHARP improvement in performance feedback in the operating room. *Annals of Surgery*, **258(6)**: 958–63.

Arora, S., Runnacles, J., Ahmed, M. *et al.* (2012) *The London handbook for debriefing: Enhancing performance debriefing in clinical and simulated settings*. Imperial College London.

Benham-Hutchins, M. and Lall, M.P. (2015) Perception of nursing education uses of Second Life by graduate nursing students. *CIN: Computers, Informatics, Nursing*, **33(9)**: 404–9.

Borneuf, A.M. and Rickels, S. (2016) *The staff nurse toolkit. Simulation proforma*: 1–73. Manchester Metropolitan University.

Department of Health (2011) *A framework for technology enhanced learning*. Department of Health. Available at: www.gov.uk/government/publications/a-framework-for-technology-enhanced-learning (accessed 18 August 2020).

Ericsson, K.A., Krampe, R.T. and Tesch-Römer, C. (1993) The role of deliberate practice in the acquisition of expert performance. *Psychological Review*, 100(3): 363.

Gaba, D.M. (2004) The future vision of simulation in health care. *BMJ Quality and Safety*, 13(Suppl 1): i2–i10.

Gough, S. and Greene, L. (2015) Introducing a regional simulated patient train-the-trainer programme and simulated patient common framework. *BMJ Simulation and Technology Enhanced Learning*, 1: A36.

Gough, S. and Greene, L. (2016) *Simulated patients in assessment*. Health Education North West.

Gough, S., Greene, L., Nestel, D. *et al.* (2015) *Simulated patients: A standardised, quality assured approach to training and implementation. Final Project Report*. Health Education North West.

Gough, S., Yohannes, A.M. and Murray, J. (2016a) The integrated simulation and technology enhanced learning (ISTEL) framework: facilitating robust design, implementation, evaluation and research in healthcare. *Physiotherapy*, 102(Suppl 1): e27–8.

Gough, S., Yohannes, A.M. and Murray, J. (2016b) Using video-reflexive ethnography and simulation-based education to explore patient management and error recognition in pre-registration physiotherapy. *Advances in Simulation*, 1(9): 1–16.

Greene, L. and Gough, S. (2016) *Simulated patients: Blending performing arts pedagogy and healthcare education. Final project report*. Health Education North West.

Greene, L., Hamshire, C., Hannan, E., Jack, K. and Wright, D.J. (2020) PG113 'Birley place': a virtual community for health and social care education. *BMJ Simulation and Technology Enhanced Learning*, 6: A94.

Grypma, S. (2012) Regarding Mrs Chase. *Journal of Christian Nursing*, 29(3): 181.

Herrmann, E.K. (1981) Mrs Chase: a noble and enduring figure. *The American Journal of Nursing*, 81(10): 1836.

Hyland, J.R. and Hawkins, M.C. (2009) High-fidelity human simulation in nursing education: A review of literature and guide for implementation. *Teaching and Learning in Nursing*, 4(1): 14–21.

International Nursing Association for Clinical Simulation and Learning (INACSL) Standards Committee (2016a) INACSL standards of best practice: Simulation[SM] simulation design. *Clinical Simulation in Nursing*, 12(S): S5–S12. Available at: https://www.inacsl.org/INACSL/document-server/?cfp=INACSL/assets/File/public/standards/SOBPEnglishCombo.pdf (accessed 18 August 2020).

International Nursing Association for Clinical Simulation and Learning (INACSL) Standards Committee (2016b) INACSL standards of best practice: Simulation^SM simulation glossary. *Clinical Simulation in Nursing,* **12(S):** S39–47. Available at: www.nursingsimulation.org/article/S1876-1399(16)30133-5/pdf (accessed 30 November 2020).

Jaye, P., Thomas, L. and Reedy, G. (2015) 'The Diamond': A structure for simulation debrief. *The Clinical Teacher,* **12(3):** 171–5.

Kolb, D.A. (1984) *Experiential learning: Experience as the source of learning and development.* Volume 1. Prentice-Hall.

Linden Research, Inc. (2019) Available at: www.lindenlab.com/about (accessed 18 August 2020).

Lioce, L. (Ed.), Lopreiato, J. (Founding Ed.), Downing, D., Chang, T.P., Robertson, J.M., Anderson, M., Diaz, D.A., and Spain, A.E. (Assoc. Eds) and the Terminology and Concepts Working Group (2020), *Healthcare Simulation Dictionary* (2nd edition). Agency for Healthcare Research and Quality.

Müller, M., Jürgens, J., Redaèlli, M. *et al.* (2018) Impact of the communication and patient hand-off tool SBAR on patient safety: a systematic review. *BMJ Open,* **8(8):** e022202.

Nehring, W.M. and Lashley, F.R. (2009) Nursing simulation: A review of the past 40 years. *Simulation and Gaming,* **40(4):** 528–52.

Nestel, D., Clark, S., Ashwell, V. *et al.* (2010) Defining responsibilities of simulated patients in medical education. *Simulation in Healthcare,* **5:** 161–8.

Nestel, D. and Bearman, M. (2015) Introduction to simulated patient methodology. In: Nestel, D. and Bearman, M. (editors) *Simulated patient methodology: Theory, evidence and practice.* Wiley-Blackwell.

Nestel, D. and Gough, S. (2018) Educating for professional practice through simulation. In: Delany, C. and Molloy, E. (editors). *Learning and teaching in clinical contexts: A practical guide.* Elsevier, pp. 175–192.

North West Simulation Education Network (NWSEN) (2016) *Simulation proforma.* Health Education England.

Nursing and Midwifery Council (2018a) *Future nurse: Standards of proficiency for registered nurses.* NMC. Available at: www.nmc.org.uk/globalassets/sitedocuments/education-standards/future-nurse-proficiencies.pdf (accessed 17 August 2020).

Nursing and Midwifery Council (2018b) *Realising professionalism: Part 1: Standards framework for nursing and midwifery education.* NMC. Available at: www.nmc.org.uk/globalassets/sitedocuments/education-standards/education-framework.pdf (accessed 13 August 2020).

Purva, M., Baxendale, B. and Scales, E. (2016) *Simulation based education in healthcare. Standards Framework and Guidance.* Association for Simulated Practice in Healthcare (ASPiH). Available at: https://aspih.org.uk/wp-content/uploads/2017/10/ASPiH-Standards-Second-version.Feb-2016.pdf (accessed 23 November 2020)

Roberts, D. (2010) Vicarious learning: a review of the literature. *Nurse Education in Practice*, 10(1): 13–16.

Roberts, D. and Greene, L. (2011) The theatre of high-fidelity simulation education. *Nurse Education Today*, 31(7): 694–8.

Schaffer, M.A., Tiffany, J.M., Kantack, K. and Anderson, L.J. (2016) Second Life® virtual learning in public health nursing. *Journal of Nursing Education*, 55(9): 536–40.

Skinner, B.F. (1938) *The behavior of organisms: an experimental analysis.* Appleton Century.

Smith, C.M., O'Byrne, C.C. and Nestel, D. (2015) Simulated patient methodology and assessment. In: Nestel, D. and Bearman, M. (editors) *Simulated patient methodology: Theory, evidence and practice.* Wiley Blackwell.

Stewart, K.R. and Hand, K.A. (2017) SBAR, communication, and patient safety: An integrated literature review. *MedSurg Nursing*, 26(5): 297–305.

Sutherland, I.E. (1968) A head-mounted three dimensional display. *Proceedings of the Fall Joint Computer Conference*, 33: 757–64.

Tiffany, J. and Hoglund, B.A. (2014) Teaching/learning in Second Life: Perspectives of future nurse-educators. *Clinical Simulation in Nursing*, 10(1): e19–e24.

Topol, E. (2019) *The Topol review: Preparing the healthcare workforce to deliver the digital future: An independent report on behalf of the Secretary of State for Health and Social Care.* Available at: https://topol.hee.nhs.uk/wp-content/uploads/HEE-Topol-Review-2019.pdf (accessed 18 August 2020).

Walia, N., Zahedi, F.M. and Jain, H. (2017) Potential of virtual worlds for nursing care: Lessons and outcomes. *Online Journal of Issues in Nursing*, 23(1).

ACTIVITY ANSWER GUIDE

ACTIVITY 8.1

Clinical and non-clinical skills that students should learn while working with you, or knowledge that you expect students to have before they arrive:

	Clinical skills	Non-psychomotor skills
Part 1/Year 1	Undertake and record vital signs Knowledge of normal range for children/adults for each vital sign	Make introductions to patients using the "Hello my name is ..." approach
Part 2/Year 2	Use and interpret early warning scores associated with the deteriorating patient Escalate concerns to nurse in charge	Use enhanced communication skills to describe the patient's condition to the nurse in charge and to alleviate patient anxiety
Part 3/Year 3		Show leadership and assertiveness skills in communicating concerns with the medical team to prompt appropriate action

CHAPTER 9

THE FUTURE OF PRACTICE LEARNING

Jacqueline Leigh

9.1 INTRODUCTION

This chapter explores the future of practice learning, applying the core concepts of a learning organisation to promote excellence (quality and governance); it therefore looks at the whole picture, considering strategies that enable creative thinking around innovative student learning experiences. Explored is the application of leadership knowledge and skills that when used effectively create the right environment whereby practice learning can flourish. Activities in this chapter include being introduced to a scenario about setting up a community of practice, providing opportunities to reflect, plan and develop strategies to sustain clinical practice as an effective and key environment where student learning can take place.

After reading this chapter you will be able to:

- Identify the Nursing and Midwifery Council (NMC) requirements for creating the right environment for practice learning and effective supervision and assessment
- Understand the core concepts (five disciplines) of a learning organisation and how these can be used to sustain clinical practice as an effective and key environment where student learning takes place
- Explore what is meant by leadership and how leadership skills can be applied to create opportunities for innovative practice learning and to promote the quality practice learning environment
- Consider strategies that enable creative thinking around innovative student learning experiences, such as social prescribing and those that take place outside traditional healthcare organisations.

In 2018 the NMC launched its *Future nurse: Standards of proficiency for registered nurses* (NMC, 2018a). First introduced to you in *Chapter 1,* these standards specify the knowledge and skills that NMC registrants must demonstrate when caring for people of all ages and across all care settings. They reflect what the public expect nurses to know and be able to do to ensure the delivery of safe, compassionate and effective care.

Also published in 2018, the *Realising professionalism* standards for education and training (NMC, 2018b, c, d) include *Part 1: Standards framework for nursing and midwifery education* (NMC, 2018b), *Part 2: Standards for student supervision and assessment* (NMC, 2018c), and *Part 3: Standards for education and training* specific to each approved programme (NMC, 2018d). A key message and something that maintains continuity with preceding standards is the fundamental requirement for partnerships between universities and healthcare organisations to provide the practice learning for students and to promote a culture for creating the best practice learning environment. Attenborough *et al.* (2019, p. 132) also refer to work-based learning (WBL) that represents "a transition from education that is designed by academic staff and led by higher education institutions, to education delivered in partnership, with increased collaboration between education providers and the clinical environment".

9.2 CREATING THE BEST ENVIRONMENT FOR PRACTICE LEARNING AND SUPERVISION AND ASSESSMENT

Looking critically at the NMC standards, there are clear messages that those in the university and healthcare organisation who have a responsibility for the organisation of practice learning should understand and then apply to create innovative practice learning experiences for students and to promote the effective learning environment. These are summarised below:

- Practice learning complies with the NMC standards framework for nursing and midwifery education
- Practice learning complies with specific programme standards
- Practice learning must be designed to meet proficiencies and outcomes relevant to the programme
- There are suitable systems, processes, resources and individuals in place to ensure safe and effective coordination of learning within practice learning environments
- There is a nominated person for each practice setting to actively support students and address student concerns
- Students have opportunities to learn from a range of relevant people in practice learning environments, including service users, registered and non-registered individuals, and other students as appropriate

- Learning experiences are inclusive and support the diverse needs of individual students
- Learning experiences are tailored to the student's stage of learning, proficiencies and programme outcomes
- All nurses, midwives and nursing associates contribute to practice learning in accordance with *The Code* (NMC, 2018e).

Nursing in the UK is often in the spotlight. Reasons for this include major incidents such as how the NMC supported nurses and midwives to effectively work through a pandemic. A pandemic describes an infectious disease where we see significant and ongoing person-to-person spread in multiple countries around the world at the same time. The COVID-19 pandemic brought immense challenges to the way that supervision and assessment was maintained in those clinical settings that rapidly changed to meet acutely ill patients' needs.

There have been other major incidents or situations where nurses and nursing services have had to respond quickly; for example, the bomb explosion in the MEN Arena (Manchester) following a pop concert in 2017, where 22 people died and over 50 were badly injured (many of them children).

Situations such as these also bring opportunities for students to work alongside a range of key staff delivering healthcare during challenging times where decision-making comes to the fore. Indeed, *Chapter 2* reports how the NMC part 2 standards (NMC, 2018c) have widened the supervisory role to include non-nursing and midwifery registrants, and this is now proving to be a crucial change from the previous profession-centric approach to mentorship (NMC, 2008). This welcome departure provides the platform for offering authentic interprofessional teaching and learning opportunities. Providing nursing and midwifery care in a time of crisis brings opportunities to think differently about practice learning and the environment within which teaching and learning is taking place.

In response to the COVID-19 situation, the NMC developed a number of emergency programme standards aimed to provide university and practice learning partners with the flexibility to enable students within the final 6 months of their pre-registration nursing and midwifery programmes to become part of the workforce, employed part-time (up to 80% practice/minimum 20% academic), with no supernumerary status provided (NMC, 2020a). These changes enabled students to help support the workforce and make use of the knowledge and skills that they had developed while also continuing their programme, registering with the NMC on time.

September 2020 saw the removal of the NMC emergency standards, with the NMC implementing its Recovery Standards (NMC, 2020b); however, providing students with supervision and assessment opportunities during a pandemic may become the new 'normal'. In times of crisis, the NMC worked together with all four countries in the UK and NHS Staff Council to mobilise the student healthcare workforce through creating national roles such as aspirant nurse (Health Education England, 2020; NHS Staff Council, 2020; NMC, 2020a). Taking on these roles, there are examples of students supporting patients as they died in hospital without loved ones and comforting patients crying through sadness, fear or pure exhaustion (Leigh *et al.*, 2020a). Emergent supervision and delegation frameworks provided guidance on how to supervise and assess students who were no longer supernumerary but required protected learning time (Health Education England 2020; Leigh *et al.*, 2020b; NMC, 2020a). It is perhaps pertinent to consider Eraut's 'continuum of formality' in learning (Eraut, 2004), with practice supervisors and practice assessors capitalising on the range of formal and informal leaning opportunities available to students from within the clinical learning environment. Creating and capitalising on supervision and assessment opportunities required the practice supervisor and practice assessor to delegate effectively nursing activities to the student. Equally, each student should consider all the options before accepting a role or activity delegated to them. The NMC defines delegation as: "the transfer to a competent individual, of the authority to perform a specific task in a specified situation" (NMC, 2019, p. 3).

Provided below are principles that practice supervisors and practice assessors must take account of when delegating a task or activity to the student:

- Ensure that the primary motivation for delegation is to serve the interests and needs of the patient
- Assess the degree of risk involved in the delegation
- Ensure that the delegation is appropriate, referring to the definitions and philosophies of nursing
- Consider the level of experience, proficiency, role and scope of practice of the student taking on the delegated task
- Do not delegate tasks and responsibilities that are beyond the student's proficiency to perform
- Ensure appropriate student assessment, planning, implementation, monitoring and evaluation of the delegated role/task or activity
- Communicate to the student the details of the role/task or activity in a clear, understandable way

- Decide on the level of student supervision and feedback required
- Ensure that the practice setting supports the delegation of the role/ task or activity
- Delegation of the task should be consistent with organisational policies and procedures.

Obviously the COVID-19 example is extreme but can be used as an example of how universities and healthcare organisations have needed to think creatively about practice learning, providing opportunities for effective supervision and assessment, with students learning about the roles of other disciplines and how to collaborate and interact in a team.

9.3 THE PRACTICE LEARNING ENVIRONMENT

Programmes that lead to registration with the NMC offer a range of teaching and learning strategies, recognising that learning and assessment will take place in both practice and academic settings and will involve working and learning with students from other disciplines as well as their own. This means that a proportion of the curriculum requires students to learn from within the practice learning environment. The practice learning environment therefore plays an essential part in students' learning. Researchers over the years have identified factors that promote the effective learning environment, and these include positive staff attitudes towards students, the duration of the placement, creating the right culture and atmosphere for learning, providing students with the variety of learning opportunities, and the positive student–supervisor relationship (Arkan *et al.*, 2018; Fisher and Kiernan, 2019; Jack *et al.*, 2018; Papastavrou *et al.*, 2010; Saarikoski *et al.*, 2007; Warne *et al.*, 2010). There is also classic evidence that connects the quality of nursing care with a good learning environment (Smith, 1987, 1991).

Drawing on work presented in *Chapter 2*, the importance of the gatekeeper of practice learning is evident with Ogier (1986), Fretwell (1982, 1985) and Orton (1981), as long ago as the 1980s, reporting on the role of the ward sister as the crucial person in creating the right culture for practice learning. Contemporary gatekeepers now include roles such as practice education leads who work in partnership with the practice education facilitator and the university. It would be useful for you to explore the gatekeepers within your practice learning environment.

What seems clear is that the culture of the practice learning environment is important, especially securing senior management and clinical learning environment level buy-in to ensure that practice learning and the supervision and assessment of students is taken seriously and that it is effectively resourced. Lessons can be learned from the literature reporting on the previous role of the mentor, whereby mentors reported difficulties finding time to attend preparation sessions for the role because of their heavy clinical workloads (Leigh and Roberts, 2018) with the need to develop governance systems ensuring that assessors and supervisors are prepared and supported adequately for their student-facing role. Indeed, Henderson and Eaton (2013) reported that unless a culture that establishes the value of teaching and learning in practice is fostered by senior managers, new ventures are likely to fail, whichever model of supporting clinical learning is adopted. Furthermore, Ward and McCormack (2020) suggest that the culture for learning is possible though the adoption of strategies of challenge, openness and debate.

There is the NMC expectation that universities together with their practice learning partners continuously work in partnership to consider and implement new ways to deliver practice learning and effective supervision and assessment. Introduced next is a way to create an effective practice learning environment through exploring the concepts of a learning organisation.

9.4 EXPLORING THE CONCEPTS OF A LEARNING ORGANISATION

Understanding the concepts of a learning organisation allows us to think differently about the culture required, whereby learning is valued by all people within the practice learning environment. Indeed, in *Chapter 2* an effective practice learning environment is described as requiring a learning culture that prioritises the safety of people, including patients, carers, students and educators, and enables the values of *The Code* to be upheld (NMC, 2018e).

Senge (2006, p. 3) refers to a learning organisation as one that: "continues to expand its capacity to create its future and provide opportunities and incentives for its members to learn continuously over time". People are encouraged to continually expand their capacity to create the results they desire, where new and expansive patterns of thinking are nurtured, where collective aspiration is set free, and where people are continually learning to see the whole together.

Senge (2006) identified five disciplines of a learning organisation; these are summarised in *Table 9.1* and applied to supervision, assessment and practice learning.

Table 9.1: Senge's five disciplines of a learning organisation (adapted from Senge, 2006)

Systems thinking	This relates to thinking about the whole organisation but also considering its component parts and how they interact; it involves thinking about the impact that an organisational decision may have in the short and long term; for example, the impact of reducing support for supervisor and assessor development in the short term may be negligible but in the long term impacts negatively on creating the sustainable workforce and practice learning environment
Personal mastery	Personal mastery relates to an organisation that considers individual aspirations as well as professional competence; for practice learning, supervision and assessment, lifelong learning is encouraged
Mental models	Here, people expose their own thinking to others, making clear their assumptions and by doing this it promotes a culture of openness towards new ways of thinking and learning; think about your assumptions around supervision and assessment and the practice learning environment where this is situated
Shared vision	Senge (2006, p. 9) refers to sharing a picture of the future we seek to create; this vision is shared with all members thus creating the common vision around, for example, what excellent supervision and assessment should look like for all students
Team learning	Senge (2006, p. 9) views team learning as the process of aligning and developing the capacities of a team to create the results its members truly desire; relating to supervision and assessment, a collective group of skilled practitioners are required to support students' practice learning progression towards NMC registration

9.4.1 Applying the concepts of a learning organisation to promote excellence in practice learning

Application of the concepts of a learning organisation requires support for learning from senior management. Gopee and Galloway (2014, p. 264), for example, imply that: "a learning attitude prevails in the management structures and organisational strategies". This can be seen across the UK where universities and healthcare organisations have worked in partnership to develop the systems (practice learning policies and procedures) that effectively support learning for students when undertaking programmes that lead to NMC registration. However, systems, policies and procedures alone will not create vibrant communities that provide the incentives and culture for individuals and teams to work together to re-think practice learning.

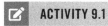 **ACTIVITY 9.1**

Consider approaches that you use that help embed the concepts of a learning organisation from within your practice learning environment. Use Senge's (2006) five disciplines introduced to you in *Table 9.1* to frame your thinking. This is a personal reflective activity, so no answer guide is provided.

What you may have considered are the positive things that are in place such as the way that your learning needs are addressed that promote mastery in supervision and assessment, met through, for example, effective personal development review. You may have identified how the overall philosophy and vision for practice learning is embedded within everybody's everyday practice. Indeed, delivering on the ambitions of the *NHS long term plan* (Department of Health and Social Care, 2019) requires a workforce (those working in a practice supervisory role) that both works in a more multidisciplinary way and includes staff who have a wider range of, or different, skills to the current mix. You may have identified the ways that you measure the effectiveness of practice learning from a student perspective and how student feedback is viewed as an opportunity for future team learning.

The NMC takes the quality of the clinical learning environment seriously, setting clear educational governance and quality standards. For example, in NMC *Part 1: Standards framework for nursing and midwifery education* the NMC expects that there are:

> "*effective governance systems that ensure compliance with all legal, regulatory, professional and educational requirements, differentiating where appropriate between the devolved legislatures of the United Kingdom, with clear lines of responsibility and accountability for meeting those requirements and responding when standards are not met, in all learning environments*". (NMC, 2018b, p. 7)

The NMC also states that all learning environments optimise safety and quality, taking account of the diverse needs of, and working in partnership with, service users, students and all other stakeholders.

It would be useful for you to find out what structures are in place to proactively identify and act on any practice learning areas for improvement, considering the role that you will play. Take, for example, student evaluations. This is one measure that the NMC and university use to demonstrate the quality of the practice learning environment. This is often measured from different perspectives such as student support, quality and student experience. Students evaluate their practice learning during or at the end of each practice learning experience. These evaluations are often submitted by students online, with the person responsible for coordinating practice learning at the placement area reviewing the results with the organisation's practice education facilitator and university. Action plans are then developed that close the loop for quality assurance. Samples of student evaluation statements are considered in *Table 9.2*.

Table 9.2: *Samples of student evaluation statements*

Student support	Quality	Student experience
My practice assessment interviews were conducted at the required times during my placement (i.e. preliminary, mid-way and final point)	Sufficient preparatory information prior to my placement(s) was available	I was encouraged to contribute to the plan of care where appropriate
All sections of my practice assessment documentation were completed accurately and timely	My named practice assessor and practice supervisor or placement educator were identified prior to being on placement	I was encouraged to reflect on practice learning experiences
I received regular and timely feedback on my performance throughout my placement	Practice learning opportunities were identified and relevant to my current stage in the programme of study	I am satisfied with my placement experience
I received constructive verbal and written feedback on my performance throughout my placement	My learning needs were recognised, and help was offered with attainment of outcomes, action plans and goals	
I was supported and encouraged to work within my personal and professional scope of practice relevant to my current stage in the programme of study	I was encouraged to undertake a range of learning activities relevant to my stage in the programme of study	
I felt supported throughout my placement by my practice education facilitator/mentor/educator and academic link in practice	I was able to achieve my placement learning outcomes	
Staff were keen to facilitate and supervise my learning activities	I was given my shifts/hours of work for the first week before my placement began	

Explored next is how applying leadership skills can create opportunities for innovative practice learning and promote the quality practice learning environment (educational governance and quality).

9.5 APPLYING LEADERSHIP SKILLS TO CREATE OPPORTUNITIES FOR INNOVATIVE PRACTICE LEARNING AND TO PROMOTE THE QUALITY PRACTICE LEARNING ENVIRONMENT

While leadership is a prominent feature in both the *NHS long term plan* (Department of Health and Social Care, 2019) and the *We Are The NHS: People plan 2020/21 – action for us all* (NHSi, 2020), leadership can be a difficult concept to understand and this is because it comes with many definitions. For example, leadership is often defined through describing observed behaviours demonstrated by the leader (Barr and Dowding, 2019), a process that motivates people, or whereby an individual influences others to achieve a common purpose. Chadwick and Leigh (2018, p. 119) define leadership as "influencing and motivating others to work effectively and to meet the goals and objectives of the service and the wider organisation". There is a link between leadership and management; however, the key function of management is to provide order and consistency to practice learning, whereas the primary function of leadership is to innovate and promote movement.

Universities and practice partners must apply exemplary leadership skills to secure innovative approaches to practice learning and to maintain quality and consistency of supervision and assessment, thinking creatively about practice learning and how to involve other disciplines in the supervision of students in the practice setting – ensuring that every student is treated as an individual.

✎ ACTIVITY 9.2

Think about a person that you have worked with or currently work with who positively influences practice learning, supervision and assessment. List the leadership qualities or behaviours that this person demonstrates.
This is a personal reflective activity, so no answer guide is provided.

It would be interesting to understand the person that you have been thinking about when engaging with *Activity 9.2*, such as the qualities and behaviours that they demonstrate. An important concept to consider, when thinking about leadership and practice learning, is that a person does not need to be in a perceived position of power to be a leader. For example, the matron is automatically viewed as a leader due to their title and job role. Practice supervisors and practice assessors are also leaders. This is due to the influence that they have over creating the culture for practice learning and through role modelling (Johnson, 2015) the right behaviours for supervision and assessment such as conducting the timely and evidence-based assessments and understanding the learning needs of individual students. In other words, we can all lead through the power of influence and not through the position of power – even if we do not have a formal leadership role.

There is no consensus in the evidence base as to the best or most important qualities and behaviours required by the effective leader. Contemporary evidence points towards inclusive and compassionate leadership. De Brún *et al.* (2019), for example, apply inclusive leadership to promote the productive work environment (or learning environment), while Zeng *et al.* (2020) link inclusive leadership to an individt growth. The compassionate leader actively supports the te through the challenges faced, demonstrating empathy (West Crucial to creating the practice learning opportunities is leaders of practice learning to empower, enthuse, challenge staff to realise the role they play in creating the best prac environment, and identify and support individual student le Frontline educational leaders such as practice supervisors, pra and practice education facilitators are required to champion practice learning, and they play a crucial role in developi workforce. Educational leaders need to be able to embrac demonstrate innovative and creative approaches to work thr educational leadership and management situations, with confidence. Kouses and Posner (2017), for example, offer th of exemplary leadership that can be applied to the practice le (see *Table 9.3*).

Table 9.3: Five practices of exemplary leadership, as applied to the practice (adapted from Kouses and Posner, 2017)

Model the way	Role model those behaviours that set th practice learning (behaviours reflect sh
Inspire a shared vision	Have a clear vision as to what exemplar looks like and share this vision from the
Challenge the process	Seek out the opportunities that provid innovative practice learning experienc afraid to challenge the status quo or p
Enable others to act	Be collaborative, enable and empowe
Encourage the heart	Celebrate and recognise each and eve to the student's learning

The healthcare leadership model (NHS Leadership Aca useful tool to explore because it describes the things yor doing at work daily, and demonstrates how you can de even if you are not in a formal leadership role.

ACTIVITY 9.3

Access the following link to download and familiarise yourself healthcare leadership model: www.leadershipacademy.nhs.ul uploads/2014/10/NHSLeadership-LeadershipModel-colour.pd
No answer guide is required for this activity.

ble 9.4: Summary of the healthcare leadership dimensions and impact on quality
hancement

ealthcare leadership imension	What does it mean for the organisation of practice learning and for promoting the quality practice learning environment?
spiring shared purpose	Leaders create a shared purpose for the collective and range of people who have a vested interest in creating and sustaining the quality practice learning environment; it is the inspiring of the shared values that is key
ading with care	Leaders behave in a way that demonstrates that they care for their practice learning team; helping to manage unsettling feelings means that energy is focused on delivering innovative practice learning
aluating information	Leaders can seek out information that is then used to maintain or create opportunities for new ways of working. Key information relates to, for example, NMC quality and governance frameworks such as practice learning audit and student evaluations; investigating what is happening is a key leadership behaviour
nnecting our service	Leaders understand how different services connect and the implications on student supervision and assessment; leaders also understand how things are done in different teams and organisations and this understanding is important when providing students with innovative practice learning experiences; for example, leaders are aware of those opportunities that will enhance the students' learning; an example is the student on an acute stroke placement provided with the opportunity to work with community groups such as Manchester Stroke Recovery Service, or organisations that assess home environments in Wales
ring the vision	Leaders can paint a picture of what quality practice learning looks like and what everyone should be working towards; this ensures that everyone is moving in the same direction, helping each person to see how their work fits
aging the team	Leaders create a culture that recognises the importance of teamwork; they value each and everybody's contribution to developing the practice learning environment; the culture and atmosphere promote staff engagement and the sharing of ideas
ding to account	Leaders hold people to account for their actions and responsibilities and this in turn drives up practice learning standards; there is a clear and agreed consensus of what constitutes success
eloping capability	Leaders champion learning and development and promote the best environment whereby those who supervise and assess students are suitably prepared; there is a culture that appreciates the capability of its team members to develop the future workforce and supports the creation of the right systems for education and development; there is a culture that learns from successes and failure
encing for results	Leaders build relationships with people that help build future collaboration and partnerships; this is important as the NMC recognises the partnerships required between healthcare organisations and the university when delivering practice learning for NMC future registrants; resources are then allocated appropriately

The model is made up of nine leadership dimensions. Do take th explore each dimension and do think about your own leadership b and those behaviours that you would expect others to demons influence practice learning. Important to know is how the mod equally to the whole variety of roles and care settings that ex healthcare and this includes student-facing education roles.

Once you have explored the nine dimensions you may hav that a key feature of the behaviours is about people working c Through empowering others to work differently within a practice learning environment, good leaders are better able to provide a vision for the future of their organisations. Indeed H (2016) report how better outcomes can be delivered by engagi teams in reducing variations and changing the way care is deliv concept can be applied to reducing variations in the quality learning and supervisory and assessment opportunities. Tean working together are often described in terms specific to leade as shared, distributed and collective leadership. Shared lead example, is where an activity such as the organisation of practi is shared between members of the team. Distributed leadersh on healthy relationships between people and used to effective a specific practice learning related activity. Collective leader reliant on everyone taking responsibility for the success of the c as a whole and not just for their own jobs or work area (2015). Take the student evaluation of practice learning as i The evaluations are reviewed by education leaders at the un healthcare organisation. Collectively, action plans are put manage any issues identified.

Offered in *Table 9.4* is a summary of each of the healthca nine dimensions together with an example of what they n organisation of practice learning and for promoting the qua learning environment.

☑ **ACTIVITY 9.4**

Now that you are more familiar with the healthcare leadership mo nine dimensions, you may wish to complete the free self-assessme helps you to assess your leadership behaviours and more fully und leadership development needs: www.leadershipacademy.nhs.uk/r healthcare-leadership-model/supporting-tools-resources/healthc leadership-model-self-assessment-tool/

ACTIVITY 9.4   *(cont'd)*

There is also the 360-degree feedback tool that will provide you with further insight into other people's perceptions of your leadership abilities and behaviour. This feedback opportunity has a cost implication so do discuss with your line manager if you feel that this is a useful tool to engage with: www.leadershipacademy.nhs.uk/resources/healthcare-leadership-model/ supporting-tools-resources/healthcare-leadership-model-360-degree-feedback-tool/

No answer guide is required for this activity.

6 APPLYING THE CONCEPTS (FIVE DISCIPLINES) OF A LEARNING ORGANISATION TOGETHER WITH THE QUALITIES AND BEHAVIOURS OF THE LEADER TO PROMOTE EFFECTIVE PRACTICE LEARNING

»xt you are asked to think about utilising the concepts (five disciplines) a learning organisation (previously summarised in *Table* 9.3) together th the qualities and behaviours of the leader to promote effective practice rning. To help you do this *Scenario 9.1* has been developed. You are ‹ed to read the scenario and then complete *Activity 9.5*.

SCENARIO 9.1

Nightingale University and its partner practice healthcare organisations have decided to work collectively and as a team to create a 'community of practice' to explore innovative ways to promote the effective practice learning environment and supervision and assessment.

The practice education facilitator from the healthcare organisation together with the university link lecturer are conscious that communities of practice will be new to most people so they provide the definition from the outset, reporting it as an organised group of professional people who share the same interests in resolving an issue, improving skills and learning from each other's experiences. They have summarised top tips for the effective implementation and sustainability of communities of practice and share this at an initial team meeting under the agenda item of the quality learning environment for students.

9.6.1 Tips for the effective implementation and sustainability of communities of practice

1. Have a clear objective or purpose of the community of practice from the outset
2. Think about who should attend, and the experience and knowledge that each person brings to the community
3. Establish infrastructures: communication methods, how often to meet, consider face-to-face or virtual meetings, what are the expectations for the community
4. Hold the initial meeting for all members
5. Consider the facilitator or chair to moderate
6. Consider social media platforms to spread the word and keep in touch

Moving forward the team has agreed to implement the community of practice concept through the setting up of a practice learning forum.

 ACTIVITY 9.5

What would your terms of reference be for the practice learning forum? Use the above Top tips when considering your answer.
An answer guide is provided at the end of this chapter.

9.7 APPLYING STRATEGIES FOR CREATING INNOVATIVE STUDENT LEARNING EXPERIENCES

The next part of this chapter considers ways to think creatively about innovative student learning experiences, such as social prescribing and those that take place outside traditional healthcare organisations.

The NMC is clear that those educational leaders in the university and healthcare organisation who have a responsibility for the organisation of practice learning should create innovative practice learning experiences for students. One way to be creative is to use a results-orientated strategic planning approach. This sounds complicated but this approach can be used at the individual practice learning (placement) level by a group of practice supervisors and practice assessors, across organisation directorates such as medicine or surgery, organisation wide, or even multi-organisational when, for example, following the patient or student's practice learning journey. There is no reason why the approach cannot be used within the voluntary, community and social enterprise (VCSE) sector, especially to explore supervision and assessment in areas that traditionally do not have an NMC nurse registrant on site.

At the centre of a results-orientated strategic planning approach is the SWOT analysis.

SWOT stands for strengths, weaknesses, opportunities and threats. A SWOT analysis is a technique that can be used for assessing these four aspects of your practice learning environment and leads to fact-based analysis, fresh perspectives and new ideas and subsequent innovations. Strengths and weaknesses are internal to your organisation and are things that you have control of and can change. Examples include who is involved with practice learning, organisational decisions, policies and procedures. Opportunities and threats are things happening outside your organisation, such as competitors or national policy. You can take advantage of opportunities and protect against threats.

Completing the SWOT analysis helps you to make the most of what you have got and then use it to your advantage by understanding what you are lacking, and eliminating things that would otherwise catch you unawares helps to reduce failure.

To complete the SWOT analysis, you are asked to transfer the SWOT template (*Table 9.5*) onto a flip chart or share electronically via a virtual meeting.

Table 9.5: SWOT template

Strengths	Weaknesses
Opportunities	**Threats**

☑ **ACTIVITY 9.6**

Undertake a SWOT analysis of the practice learning experiences for students. There is no answer guide to this activity, but before you embark on the SWOT analysis you are asked to read and consider the tips in *Section 9.7.1* for successful completion.

9.7.1 Tips for successful completion of the SWOT analysis

1. Before starting the SWOT consider who to involve, remembering that the SWOT analysis works best when completed by diverse groups or voices within and outside the practice learning environment.
2. Apply your SWOT analysis to a specific issue, such as a practice learning goal that you would like to achieve or a problem you need to solve. Note how you can conduct separate SWOT analyses on individual issues and combine them. Further SWOTs could include issues/problems associated with student practice placement capacity, protected learning time for practice supervisors and practice assessors, or addressing the content and context of student evaluations.
3. Consider the cue questions identified for each SWOT quadrant in *Table 9.6* as a starting point but be creative and be prepared to think outside of the box.
4. Use the qualities of the effective leader to effectively challenge!
5. Keep your SWOT simple and short, including key information such as the evidence as to why you consider staff as a strength – their specific capabilities and roles performed that benefit student learning and how they can help you meet your business goals – supply chain of future NMC quality registrants (as an example).
6. Following completion of the SWOT, analyse and prioritise the results by listing or ranking them in order of the most significant factors that affect practice learning to the least.
7. Look at practice learning as it is now and consider where it might be in the future, as well as aspirations and visions for the future.
8. Importantly, think about the elements that are essential to the success of practice learning – refer to the qualities of the effective learning environment considered earlier in this chapter and the things you can

offer students that others cannot. Thinking about these elements helps provide the evidence of your unique selling point and competitive advantage: the things that set your learning environment apart from others, or are unique to where you work.

Table 9.6: Questions to help complete the SWOT analysis

Strengths	What do you do particularly well? What is your unique selling point (distinguishes you from your competitors)? What advantages do you have over others (staff motivation, skills, values)? What do others see as your strengths? What brings you the clear advantage?
Weaknesses	Be honest! What can be improved (people, resources, systems and procedures)? What could be avoided? Where do you have fewer resources than others?
Opportunities	What opportunities can you exploit (think horizon scanning, national policy)? What are interesting trends? How can you turn strengths into opportunities?
Threats	What obstacles are you facing? What are the threats to practice learning from the outside (external to your organisation)? What are your competitors doing? How exposed are you to external challenges and impact on practice learning? What threats do your weaknesses expose you to?

Completing the SWOT analysis provides the opportunity for teams to think differently, brainstorming to identify the key issues. It might be that you have horizon scanned and explored contemporary healthcare and professional policy. You may have spent time together understanding the *NHS long term plan* (Department of Health and Social Care, 2019) and by doing this you can apply the key messages to promoting innovative learning experiences for students that have a public health focus such as social prescribing (Howarth and Leigh, 2020). Through interested teams exploring an issue in depth and within its context, the NMC *Part 2: Standards for student supervision and assessment* (NMC, 2018c) may be viewed as an opportunity, promoting new ways for the range of healthcare professionals to supervise students in a diverse range of setting such as the VCSE sector. While exploring an issue you may uncover strengths and opportunities; you may also uncover challenging weaknesses and threats. Continuing with the example of providing student learning experiences from within the VCSE sector, these weaknesses and threats may relate to the availability of practice assessors in organisations that do not traditionally have an NMC registrant on site. This is where conducting a further SWOT analysis specifically around supervision and assessment in the VCSE sector will help you keep finding solutions to problems and to consistently innovate practice learning opportunities for students. Adopting this inquisitive and problem-solving approach, the team are demonstrating key leadership behaviours and indeed transforming practice learning from within a culture of a learning organisation.

9.8 ALTERNATIVE MODELS OF NURSE EDUCATION

Considered in this final part of the chapter are alternative models of nurse education. Utilising the SWOT analysis and through applying leadership behaviours to think differently about practice learning, new models of nurse education may begin to emerge. An example includes thinking about service learning models whereby students on placement are intentionally viewed as an asset to the service (or organisation) and whereby the learning enhances the service (Clayton *et al.*, 2010; Mason and Dunens, 2019). Giles and Eyler (1994) and Pacho (2015) propose the theoretical roots of service learning in John Dewey's work that reports on learning from experience, reflective activity, citizenship, community and democracy (Dewey, 1916, 1938).

A similar mindset links back to the notion of nursing development units, which were first mooted in the UK in the early 1980s and where the emphasis was on becoming a place where innovative nursing practice was fostered, where practice was scrutinised and evaluated and where clinicians were active researchers. Since then, the term practice development unit appears to have evolved, but the principles remain largely unchanged. Page (2002) argues that there has been growing emphasis on defining standards of practice, implementing evidence-based practice and encouraging innovation in organisations and clinical teams. Indeed, the NMC is clear in its standards for supervision and assessment that all students are provided with safe, effective and inclusive learning (NMC, 2018c, p. 6).

Across the UK, several academic centres have developed that provide potential practice development units with opportunities to be formally assessed against specific criteria and subsequently accredited for their development; for example, Bournemouth, Leeds and Swansea universities. Gerrish (2001) evaluated practice development units accredited by a single centre and found that factors leading to successful units included the role of the clinical leader, motivation of the unit members themselves, financial resources and buy-in from senior managers and doctors. Many of the success factors link to the need for collective and shared leadership and to the concepts of the learning organisation (Senge, 2006).

Thinking differently and to the future of practice learning, we propose the development of closer clinical academic partnerships based on the Australian model outlined by Walsh *et al.* (2012) which adopts a broader interpretation of nursing knowledge in order to systematically create an area where nursing knowledge is created and extended; we term these areas 'academy areas': an innovative adjunct to supporting practice learning, building on the concept of service learning. Academy areas are characterised by a clear commitment to interprofessional practice learning, the presence of highly skilled committed healthcare professionals who actively seek out teaching opportunities with learners, and a track record of person-centred practice and associated development. Indeed this interprofessional education mindset is akin to NMC thinking around the expanded role of healthcare professionals who can supervise aspiring NMC registrants from within the practice learning environment. Previous work raises concerns that due to increasing student numbers and professional body requirements, current models of supporting clinical learning for student nurses are unsustainable (Andrews *et al.*, 2010; Lobo *et al.*, 2014), prompting educators and clinicians to develop new approaches. Ironside *et al.* (2014, p. 190) reveal that there is perhaps an overriding emphasis on task completion within practice learning which does little to foster the "more complex aspects of nursing practice such as clinical reasoning, delegation and quality improvement". One could argue that coaching models introduced in *Chapter 3* go some way to reversing this. Excitingly, our new idea of academy areas ensures that peer and facilitative learning takes place from within a practice learning environment that promotes person-centred care and whereby students are viewed as an asset. Service learning is embedded through embracing the concepts of the learning organisation, using collective and shared leadership to develop the right culture where practice supervision and practice assessment can flourish.

In the future, patients might elect to be cared for in an academy area. Academy area status would be highly prized and sought after; such is the reverence for nurse education and learning to be a nurse.

We encourage new models of nurse education to be considered; perhaps nurse education should include 2 years of theory (supported by simulated learning), a third year spent in a supernumerary capacity focusing on learning with more experienced colleagues, and a final internship year where the student is still learning but is paid for the contribution to the care delivery team? This final year would ease the transition to registered nurse status.

9.9 SUMMARY

This chapter has explored the future of practice learning, applying the core concepts of a learning organisation to promote excellence (quality and governance). Considering and applying strategies that enable creative thinking around innovative student learning experiences means that clinical practice continues as an effective and key environment where student learning takes place. Thinking about a person who positively influences practice learning, supervision and assessment generated a list of leadership qualities or behaviours that set the right culture where practice learning can flourish. Furthermore, applying the concepts of shared and collective leadership ensures that practice learning becomes everybody's business and that people do not need to be in a position of power to positively influence practice learning. Finally, thinking about alternative models of nurse education should be encouraged, and offered in this chapter is the idea of academy areas that embed service learning to view students as assets from within the practice learning environment.

Think about the pipeline for registered nurses and the transition of students to registered nurses: what if we were to create a perfect nurse education curriculum with practice learning experiences (something that is currently elusive)? If universities and their healthcare partners were not constrained by student fees and capped numbers, by EU regulations and when securing practice learning opportunities for first- and second-year students, consider what could be done with nurse education. Risks would have to be taken but there would be great possibilities if we were able to be bold and brave with our curriculum. Roberts and Leigh (2020) offer their thoughts around these future curriculum possibilities. Recommendations that they make in their paper include having a clear vision for nursing – being bold about the role of the nurse and being clear about the future of nursing and practice learning opportunities.

RECOMMENDED FURTHER READING

Storey, J. and Holti, R. (2013) *Towards a new model of leadership for the NHS*. London: NHS Leadership Academy. Available at: www.leadershipacademy.nhs.uk/wp-content/uploads/2013/05/Towards-a-New-Model-of-Leadership-2013.pdf (accessed 18 August 2020).

Find out more information about the NHS leadership model at: www. leadershipacademy.nhs.uk/resources/healthcare-leadership-model/
Find out more about the SWOT analysis from the Mind Tools link: www.mindtools.com/pages/article/newTMC_05.htm

REFERENCES

Andrews, M., Brewer, M., Buchan, T. *et al.* (2010) Implementation and sustainability of the nursing and midwifery standards for mentoring in the UK. *Nurse Education in Practice*, **10**: 251–5.

Arkan, B., Ordin, Y. and Yılmaz, D. (2018) Undergraduate nursing students' experience related to their clinical learning environment and factors affecting to their clinical learning process. *Nurse Education in Practice*, **29**: 127–32.

Attenborough, J., Abbott, S., Brook, J. and Knight, R.A. (2019) Everywhere and nowhere: Work-based learning in healthcare education. *Nurse Education in Practice*, **36**: 132–8.

Barr, J. and Dowding, L. (2019) *Leadership in health care.* 4th edition. Sage.

Chadwick, A. and Leigh, J.A. (2018) Identifying and developing clinical leadership in relation to transition. In: Darvill A., Stephens M. and Leigh, J.A. (editors) *Transition to nursing practice.* Sage.

Clayton, P., Bringle, R.G., Senor, B., Huq, J. and Morrison, M. (2010) Differentiating and assessing partnerships in service-learning and civic engagement: exploitative, transactional, or transformational. *Michigan Journal of Community Service Learning*, **16**: 5–22.

De Brún, A., O'Donovan, R. and McAuliffe, E. (2019) Interventions to develop collectivistic leadership in healthcare settings: a systematic review. *BMC Health Services Research*, **19**: 72.

Department of Health and Social Care (2019) *NHS long term plan.* Department of Health and Social Care.

Dewey, J. (1916/2011) *Democracy and education.* Simon and Brow.

Dewey, J. (1938) *Experience and education.* Simon and Schuster.

Eraut, M. (2004) Informal learning in the workplace. *Studies in Continuing Education*, **26**(2): 247–73. doi: 10.1080/ 158037042000225245

Fisher, M. and Kiernan, M. (2019) Student nurses' lived experience of patient safety and raising concerns, *Nurse Education Today*, **77**: 1–5.

Fretwell, J.E. (1982*) Ward teaching and learning.* Royal College of Nursing.

Fretwell, J.E. (1985) *Freedom to change: The creation of the ward learning environment.* Royal College of Nursing.

Gerrish, K. (2001) A pluralistic evaluation of nursing/practice development units. *Journal of Clinical Nursing,* **10**: 109–18.

Giles, D.E. and Eyler, J. (1994) The theoretical roots of service-learning in John Dewey: Toward a theory of service-learning. *Michigan Journal of Community Service Learning,* **1(1)**: 77–85.

Gopee, N. and Galloway, J. (2014) *Leadership and management in healthcare.* Sage.

Ham, C., McKenna, H. and Dunn, P. (2016) *Tackling the growing crisis in the NHS.* The King's Fund. Available at: www.kingsfund.org.uk/publications/articles/nhs-agenda-for-action (accessed 18 August 2020).

Health Education England (2020) *Standard operating procedure for the deployment of nursing and midwifery students in the North West of England.* Health Education England.

Henderson, A. and Eaton, E. (2013) Assisting nurses to facilitate student and new graduate learning in practice settings: What 'support' do nurses at the bedside need? *Nurse Education in Practice,* **13**: 197–201.

Howarth, M.L. and Leigh, J.A. (2020) Social prescribing: collaboration in times of stability and crisis. *British Journal of Nursing,* **29(10)**: 578–9.

Ironside, P., McNelis, A.M. and Ebright, P. (2014) Clinical education in nursing: Rethinking learning in practice settings. *Nursing Outlook,* **62(3)**: 185–91.

Jack, K., Hamshire, C., Harris, W.E. *et al.* (2018) "My mentor didn't speak to me for the first four weeks": Perceived unfairness experienced by nursing students in clinical practice settings. *Journal of Clinical Nursing,* **27(5–6)**: 929–38. doi: 10.1111/jocn.14015

Johnson, J.A. (2015) Nursing professional development specialists as role models. *Journal for Nurses in Professional Development,* **31(5)**: 297–9.

Kouses, J.M. and Posner, B.Z. (2017) *The leadership challenge: How to make extraordinary things happen in organizations.* 6th edition. Wiley.

Leigh, J.A., Bolton, M., Cain, K. *et al.* (2020a) Nursing on the frontline during the COVID-19 pandemic – reflections from student nurses, newly qualified graduate nurses and personal tutors. *British Journal of Nursing,* **29(13)**: 788–9.

Leigh, J.A., Bulpitt, S., Dunn, J. *et al.* (2020b) A guide to the NMC emergency standards for nurse education during the current deployment of student nurses. *British Journal of Nursing*, **29(11)**: 632–8.

Leigh, J.A. and Roberts, D. (2018) Critical exploration of the new NMC standards of proficiency for registered nurses. *British Journal of Nursing*, **27(18)**: 1068–72.

Lobo, C., Arthur, A. and Latimer, V. (2014) *Collaborative Learning in Practice (CLiP) for pre-registration nursing students*. Available at: www.charleneloboconsulting.com/wp-content/uploads/CLiP-Paper-final-version-Sept-14.pdf (accessed 13 August 2020).

Mason, M.R. and Dunens, E. (2019) Service-learning as a practical introduction to undergraduate public health: benefits for student outcomes and accreditation. *Frontiers in Public Health*, **7**: 63. doi: 10.3389/fpubh.2019.00063

NHS Leadership Academy (2014) *Healthcare leadership model*. NHS Leadership Academy. Available at: www.leadershipacademy.nhs.uk/resources/healthcare-leadership-model/ (accessed 29 September 2020).

NHSi (2020) *We Are The NHS: People plan 2020/21 – action for us all*. NHSi. Available at: www.england.nhs.uk/wp-content/uploads/2020/07/We_Are_The_NHS_Action_For_All_Of_Us_FINAL_24_08_20.pdf (accessed 13th November 2020)

NHS Staff Council (2020) *Deployment of student nurses during the COVID-19 emergency*. NHS Staff Council. Available at: www.nhsemployers.org/-/media/Employers/Documents/COVID19/NHS-Staff-Council-advice-job-descriptions-and-banding-of-nursing-students.pdf (accessed 18 August 2020).

Nursing and Midwifery Council (2008) *Standards to support learning and assessment in practice*: *NMC standards for mentors, practice teachers and teachers*. NMC. Available at: www.nmc.org.uk/globalassets/sitedocuments/standards/nmc-standards-to-support-learning-assessment.pdf (accessed 24th April 2020).

Nursing and Midwifery Council (2018a) *Future nurse: Standards of proficiency for registered nurses*. NMC. Available at: www.nmc.org.uk/globalassets/sitedocuments/education-standards/future-nurse-proficiencies.pdf (accessed 17 August 2020).

Nursing and Midwifery Council (2018b) *Realising professionalism: Part 1: Standards framework for nursing and midwifery education*. NMC. Available at: www.nmc.org.uk/globalassets/sitedocuments/education-standards/education-framework.pdf (accessed 13 August 2020).

Nursing and Midwifery Council (2018c) *Realising professionalism: Part 2: Standards for student supervision and assessment.* NMC. Available at: www.nmc.org.uk/globalassets/sitedocuments/education-standards/student-supervision-assessment.pdf (accessed 13 August 2020).

Nursing and Midwifery Council (2018d) *Realising professionalism: Part 3: Standards for education and training.* NMC. Available at: www.nmc.org.uk/globalassets/sitedocuments/education-standards/programme-standards-nursing.pdf (accessed 13 August 2020).

Nursing and Midwifery Council (2018e) *The Code: Professional standards of practice and behaviour for nurses, midwives and nursing associates.* NMC. Available at: www.nmc.org.uk/globalassets/sitedocuments/nmc-publications/nmc-code.pdf (accessed 29 September 2020).

Nursing and Midwifery Council (2019) *Delegation and accountability: supplementary information to the NMC Code.* NMC. Available at: www.nmc.org.uk/globalassets/sitedocuments/nmc-publications/delegation-and-accountability-supplementary-information-to-the-nmc-code.pdf (accessed 18 August 2020).

Nursing and Midwifery Council (2020a) *Emergency standards for nursing and midwifery education.* NMC. Available at: www.nmc.org.uk/standards-for-education-and-training/emergency-education-standards/ (accessed 13 August 2020).

Nursing and Midwifery Council (2020b) *Recovery programme standards.* NMC. Available at: www.nmc.org.uk/globalassets/sitedocuments/education-standards/recovery-programme-standards.pdf (accessed 17 December 2020).

Ogier, M.E. (1986) Sister/staff nurse and the nurse learner. *Nurse Education Today*, 6(1): 16–22.

Orton, H. (1981) *Ward learning climate.* Royal College of Nursing.

Pacho, T.O. (2015) Unpacking John Dewey's connection to service-learning. *Journal of Education and Social Policy*, 2(3): 8–16.

Page, S. (2002) The role of practice development in modernising the NHS. *Nursing Times*, 98(11): 34.

Papastavrou, E., Lambrinou, E., Tsangari, H., Saarikoski, M. and Leino-Kilpi, H. (2010) Student nurses' experience of learning in the clinical environment. *Nurse Education in Practice*, 10: 176–82.

Roberts, D. and Leigh, J. (2020) The future of nurse education: imagining the art of the possible. *British Journal of Nursing*, 29(16): 968–70.

Saarikoski, M., Marrow, C., Abreu, W., Riklikiene, O. and Özbicakci, S. (2007) Student nurses' experience of supervision and mentorship in clinical practice: a cross cultural perspective. *Nurse Education in Practice*, 7: 407–15.

Senge, P.M. (2006) *The fifth discipline: The art and practice of the learning organization.* Random House.

Smith, P. (1987) The relationship between quality of nursing care and the ward as a learning environment: developing a methodology. *Journal of Advanced Nursing*, 12: 413–20.

Smith, P. (1991) The nursing process: raising the profile of emotional care in nurse training. *Journal of Advanced Nursing*, 16: 74–81.

Walsh, K., Kitson, A., Cross, W. *et al.* (2012) A conversation about practice development and knowledge translation as mechanisms to align the academic and clinical contexts for the advancement of nursing practice. *Collegian*, 19: 67–75.

Ward, C. and McCormack, B. (2020) Creating an adult learning culture through practice development. *Nurse Education Today*, 20: 259–66.

Warne, T., Johansson, U.B., Papastavrou, E. *et al.* (2010) An exploration of the clinical learning experience of nursing students in nine European countries. *Nurse Education Today*, 30: 809–15.

West, M., Armit, K., Loewenthal, L. *et al.* (2015) *Leadership and leadership development in health care: The evidence base.* The King's Fund. Available at: www.kingsfund.org.uk/publications/ leadership-and-leadership-development-health-care (accessed 18 August 2020).

West, M., Collins, B., Eckert, R. and Chowla, R. (2017) *Caring to change. How compassionate leadership can stimulate innovation in health care.* The King's Fund. Available at: www.kingsfund.org.uk/ publications/caring-change (accessed 18 August 2020).

Zeng, H., Zhao, L. and Zhao, Y. (2020) Inclusive leadership and taking-charge behavior: Roles of psychological safety and thriving at work. *Frontiers in Psychology*, 11(62): 1–11.

ACTIVITY ANSWER GUIDE

ACTIVITY 9.5

Provided below is an exemplar terms of reference for a practice learning forum that applies the evidence for effective communities of practice.

Practice learning forum terms of reference

Constitution

The practice learning forum is a collaborative group of professionals from both a university and its partner practice learning healthcare organisations. With a shared passion and expertise in the field of practice learning, the group acts as a community of practice and forum for collaboration, governance and innovation.

Core business

- Maintain an effective communications framework between university and practice learning partners
- Quality assurance/practice governance for undergraduate nursing and trainee nursing associate approved programmes of education
- Influence and support decision-making around practice learning matters
- Forum for the development of innovative practice learning

Membership

- Practice learning lead: (chair)
- Director of placements (quality assurance and enhancement)
- Director of health
- Student placement administrator
- Partner healthcare organisation education leads
- Practice education facilitator representation from partner practice learning organisations
- Undergraduate programme leader representation
- University link lecturer lead representation

Responsibilities of members of the group

All members of the group should ensure effective dissemination of information and any programmes of work within their own organisation.

Frequency of meetings

Meetings will occur every 2 months, to be reviewed after 6 months. Any 'task & finish' groups will meet as required.

The meeting will be chaired by the Professor of Nurse Education. Notes of the meeting will be taken and shared with the group.

For the group to be quorate it should have the following representatives:
- Chair
- At least two practice learning representatives
- At least two university representatives with programme responsibilities.

Reporting arrangements

The practice learning forum will work collaboratively, reporting to university and practice learning partners' organisational groups/committees. Additionally, the forum will be responsible for ensuring outputs are appropriately shared across all localities.

Review

The Terms of Reference will be reviewed in September 2021.

INDEX